OXFORD MEDICAL PUBLICATIONS

Basic Medical Education

Basic Medical Education

DAVID SINCLAIR, M.A., M.D., D.SC., F.R.C.S.Ed.

Regius Professor of Anatomy, University of Aberdeen

LONDON
OXFORD UNIVERSITY PRESS
1972

Oxford University Press, Ely House, London W. 1

GLASGOW NEWYORK TORONTO MELBOURNE WELLINGTON
CAPE TOWN IBADAN NAIROBI DAR ES SALAAM LUSAKA ADDIS ABABA
DELHI BOMBAY CALCUTTA MADRAS KARACHI LAHORE DACCA
KUALA LUMPUR SINGAPORE HONG KONG TOKYO

ISBN 0 19 264913 2

© Oxford University Press 1972

Set in Great Britain by Gloucester Typesetting Co. Ltd
and printed by The Camelot Press Ltd
London and Southampton

Contents

It must be considered that there is nothing more difficult to carry out, nor more doubtful of success, nor more dangerous to handle, than to initiate a new order of things. For the reformer has enemies in all those who profit by the old order, and only lukewarm defenders in all those who would profit by the new.

Machiavelli

Preface

The title of this book is the term applied by the General Medical Council to the preclinical, clinical, and preregistration periods of study in the medical schools under its jurisdiction. This phase of medical education has for a long time been subjected to much criticism and analysis, and in the last few years to considerable changes in content and organization.

In 1953, when I visited America to study trends of medical education, a wave of curricular reform was just breaking over the heads of the medical schools in the United States. At this time there was little British interest in the subject, although some schools were pioneering experimental arrangements and methods. But since 1957, when the General Medical Council relaxed the rigidity of its control over the curriculum, nearly every British medical school has been debating its own particular proposals for reform. In 1968 a further stimulus to discussion was added in the shape of the *Report of the Royal Commission on Medical Education*, which made radical suggestions regarding the undergraduate curriculum.

Members of planning or curriculum committees often have little time in which to examine critically the fundamental concepts behind the specific proposals before them, and the literature is now becoming both voluminous and diffuse. Yet virtually all the variations on the theme of medical education derive from the same basic ideas, and most of the differences between systems are due to differences in the way in which these ideas are translated into action. I therefore hope that this attempt to survey critically the foundations of curricular reform may be of interest to those who are engaged in teaching or learning in medical schools.

Although I have been a member of several planning and curriculum committees, both in Britain and in Australia, the views I have expressed must not be taken as indicating the attitude of any particular medical school or other body. Indeed, I imagine that many of my colleagues would wish to take strong exception to some of them! Nevertheless, I hope that I have been able to steer a reasonably objective course between the twin pitfalls of quarrelsome polemicism and uncritical acceptance.

I should like to thank Miss D. Marshall and Miss A. Duncan for their help with the typing of the manuscript.

Aberdeen   D.C.S.
December 1971

PART ONE

Background

I Orthodox Medical Education in Britain

> To consider medical education realistically and effectively is to consider it historically.
>
> *Edwin Clarke*

HISTORY

In order to examine the ideas and prejudices of those who at present seek to change the shape and substance of British medical education, it is necessary to begin by establishing what it is that they would like to alter. There is no better way to do this than by sketching a brief summary of the manner in which our current orthodoxy has developed, particularly in the last 100 years or so. Only a brief survey of this evolution can be given here, but further details will be found in the papers of Clarke (1966) and Cohen (1968).

Medical education is not static; it constantly changes in response to social circumstances and the needs of medical practice. In the medical schools of Britain and the Commonwealth the concept of a uniform 'official' education for doctors is only just over 100 years old, and previous to this time most students learned their trade by a form of apprenticeship.

The first British medical qualifications were given by Oxford and Cambridge, but they were very different from their modern counterparts. In 1549, during the reign of Edward VI, new statutes for the University of Oxford laid down that a medical student must study 6 years, dispute twice, respond once, and see two anatomical dissections before he obtained his B.A. Before he was admitted to practice, he had himself to perform two dissections, and also to prove that he had effected at least three cures. For his doctorate, he had to see two or three more dissections, dispute twice, and respond twice (Sinclair and Robb-Smith, 1950).

Two things are at once striking about this; the time taken to obtain the first degree is almost exactly the same as it is now, and the only scientific subject specified is anatomy. At this time anatomy *was* the only science, and the objective of the curriculum (if we may call it that) was to produce a graduate educated in the classics, with a certain amount of technical information thrown in. The 6 years were therefore spent very largely in reading and in conversation, with virtually no practical or clinical work.

This attitude towards medical education was still prevalent at the beginning of the nineteenth century. When Sir Benjamin Brodie was consulted about the education of Henry Acland, he said, 'Send the boy to Oxford, and let him pay no attention to his future profession, but do as he would if he were going into Parliament. . . . When he has taken his degree, send him to me and I will tell him what to do next' (Atlay, 1903). At this time the licensing of physicians and surgeons to practise was chaotic, and the examinations demanded very little knowledge of the practice of medicine. The licensing of physicians was in the hands of the Royal College of Physicians, but with an Oxford or Cambridge university degree a graduate could practice medicine in any part of Britain except within 7 miles of the City of London.[1] To prepare himself for the examinations the candidate attended the practice of a London hospital, listened to lectures, and 'walked the wards'. Exactly what he did was a matter for the individual. The clinical side of a doctor's education was thus a haphazard matter, and could even be evaded entirely. It was possible for a Cambridge M.A. to take a doctorate in medicine without attending a hospital or any medical lectures, and without being examined in medicine (Newman, 1957).

At this time there were three main kinds of medical practitioner—physicians, surgeons, and apothecaries. Only the physicians were university graduates, and they were described by an Act of Parliament as 'profound, sad, discreet, groundedly learned and deeply studied in Physic' (Newman, 1957). They gave an opinion when consulted, but were not expected to demean themselves by using their hands; theoretical knowledge derived from the study of books was

[1] In 1556 Dr. John Caius, then President of the College, reproved the University of Oxford for conferring a medical degree on a coppersmith who had failed to satisfy the College 3 years before: 'Because of the safety of the State we admonish you when you have conferred a degree on a man without the colour or taste of philosophy, a man far too unlearned, far too ignorant, whose answers fell below the mediocrity of a child, one with nothing to recommend him but blind audacity. This is a blot upon your University which has become the refuge for these dregs of men. And this you have done without regard to the health of our dear country.'

all they needed, since most of the physical signs of illness had yet to be recognized.

The surgeons were practical men of much commoner clay (Graham-Little, 1939), whose trade developed from that of the barbers and bloodletters. From the beginning, therefore, they were accustomed to using their hands, and any theoretical knowledge they acquired was secondary. To this day the proud physicians are prone to contrast the 'art' of medicine with the 'craft' of surgery.

The apothecaries were at first shopkeepers who dealt in drugs. They were eventually permitted to prescribe, and ultimately to care for patients. For both surgeons and apothecaries the recognized type of education was an apprenticeship, and it was not until the nineteenth century was well advanced that the universities had to bother about them at all.

The situation regarding the training of medical practitioners was thus extremely confused, and the medical profession itself began to demand reform. In 1815 Parliament passed a bill which gave the London Society of Apothecaries (a body founded by Royal Charter in 1617) what amounted to a monopoly of the training of general practitioners (Anderson, 1966). This training included apprenticeship, clinical work in a hospital, and a qualifying examination. It became gradually accepted that the study of books was not sufficient for the practice of medicine, but that some instruction in basic science and some clinical experience in hospital were necessary before a student could be allowed to practise. Those who qualified in this manner began to feel that the profession should establish sound educational standards, as well as a code of ethical behaviour. At the same time, the Government progressively became more aware of the necessity for protecting the public against the activities of unqualified quacks.

What finally emerged, in the Medical Act of 1858, was the General Medical Council, a body formed to administer this Act. The Council was charged, among other things, with the duty of maintaining a Medical Register containing the names of those medical practitioners who had satisfied the Council of their professional fitness. The purpose of the Register was to ensure a common minimum standard of education among the products of the many diverse institutions—the Society of Apothecaries, the Royal Colleges of Physicians, the Royal Colleges of Surgeons, and the universities—which granted licences to practise medicine.

The Council did not, either then or subsequently, institute qualifying examinations or tests of its own; it merely decided whether or not the education provided by a given institution was 'sufficient'. In order that it should be able to arrive at such decisions, it was given power to require information from the medical schools under its jurisdiction about their courses of study, examinations, and requirements for obtaining qualification. The Council was from the beginning able to send inspectors to report on the 'professional' examinations set by the schools, but it was not until 1950 that it was empowered to inspect the schools themselves and their courses of instruction (Sinclair, 1957a). Accordingly, most of the information reaching the Council took the form of memoranda.

If any school did not measure up to the standards which the Council set, recognition could be withdrawn from it, and this in turn meant that its graduates could not be registered. This was a real inducement to reform, since unregistered practitioners were debarred from holding appointments in the public service; they could not sign legally valid certificates, and were unable to recover medical charges in a court of law.

It was also an inducement to uniformity. Although the deliberations of the Council were at first little heeded by the medical profession (Ellis, 1966b), the increasing body of medical and scientific knowledge which could be considered suitable for inclusion in a medical course brought home to doctors the desirability of having some standardization, and the recommendations of the General Medical Council became more and more those of a body empowered to enforce its decisions.

From the beginning, the Council steadfastly disclaimed any idea of imposing uniformity, but naturally it had to inform the medical schools of the sort of course which would meet its requirements, and these prescriptions were issued in a series of 'recommendations' which, because of their source, assumed more or less the force of orders: uniformity of curricula, at least in the outlines of the course, thus became inevitable.

The Council was early in conflict with the various licensing bodies (Poynter, 1966), and the original limitation of its powers to the inspection of examinations led to the placing of undue weight on the examinations which punctuated the medical curriculum. Nevertheless, it achieved a great deal in unifying the standards of medical education.

In 1861 the Council recommended a 4-year course, and material was progressively added to this as it became available. In 1867 it produced a list of 'subjects' which it proposed should be regarded as the basic minimum of knowledge for every registered medical practitioner. This list included anatomy, physiology, chemistry, materia medica, practical pharmacy, medicine, surgery, midwifery, and forensic medicine. The idea behind a course of this kind was to produce a practitioner who was 'safe' to carry out all the functions of a physician, a surgeon, and an obstetrician, and who was also able to dispense his own medicines. In 1885 the Council specified 5 years as the time necessary for a course to which physics and biology had been added (Ellis, 1966b), and gradually more and more detailed 'recommendations' were issued, indicating how much of each 'subject' should be taught, at what stage it should be studied, and how it should be examined. The student had no longer any scope for private enterprise, except in so far as he could obtain extra tuition over and above the basic course.

The idea that every graduate recognized by the Council should be able to perform satisfactorily and safely in all branches of the profession—as surgeon, pathologist, physician, obstetrician, and so on— died hard, and it was for this reason that the curriculum grew in length and in detail. Nevertheless, even in 1885, Sir Henry Acland stated that 'the several subjects . . . had become so vast in the eyes of most specializing experts that selection and abridgement must be made. It must be made, within limits, by the responsible teachers and the responsible examiners connected with the several licensing bodies, subject to the general supervision by this Court of Appeal for all' (Poynter, 1966). But it was not perhaps until the 1914 war that it became generally realized that the curriculum was not infinitely expansible, and that nobody could learn everything required for all kinds of specialist practice. The growth of knowledge thus killed the idea of the 'safe' practitioner, and his image was gradually replaced by that of the 'well-balanced graduate'.

The main difficulty presented by this image is its exact definition. If the Council had still had to deal with the 'profound, sad' physicians of a century earlier, it could readily have formulated a curriculum for their needs, but the 'well-balanced graduate' was and is essentially a vague figure, and there has been a vast amount of vague thinking about the practical details of his education. For the last 30 or 40 years the medical schools have been attempting to produce, by theoretical instruction and practical experience, a kind of undifferentiated multipotent doctor who has a grasp of basic principles (whatever they may be) sufficient to enable him, after a further period of postgraduate specialist study, to enter any branch of the profession. Since the profession includes people as diverse as medical journalists, radiotherapists, psychiatrists, and port medical officers, it is easy to imagine the arguments in the Council over the inclusion of this subject or that, the number of hours which should be devoted to them, and whether or not they should be examinable.

The growth of specialism in the late nineteenth century led, on the one hand, to a proliferation of postgraduate professional diplomas certifying competence in a particular direction over and above the minimum standards laid down by the Council. On the other, it led to the formation in the medical schools of administratively convenient 'departments', where people interested in a particular aspect of medical science and practice could share common technical facilities and co-operate with each other in advancing the 'subject' so created. One of the ways in which this advancement could be achieved was obviously to make a successful demand for time within the medical curriculum, so that students could become interested in the new speciality and use it in their practice on qualification.

By their very nature, new subjects tend to arise sporadically in a restricted number of schools, and for some considerable period following their inception not every medical school can give instruction in all of them. The Council, anxious to produce a graduate who could turn his hand to anything given an adequate period of postgraduate instruction, was therefore hampered by an inevitable diversity in the teaching capacity of the individual medical schools. In the circumstances, the detailed and uniform 'recommendations' of the Council became more and more inapplicable to the actual situation.

Meanwhile, the first of several important independent reports on medical education to be made in the twentieth century had appeared. The Haldane Commission, which reported in 1913, emphasized the need for flexibility in the curriculum and suggested the possibility of 'elective' studies [see p. 92]. The Commission also urged the institution of whole-time clinical professorial units, along the lines of those at Johns Hopkins, as recommended by Abraham Flexner in his book (1912) on European medical education.

In 1944 two other reports, those of the Royal College of Physicians and of the Goodenough Committee, were published, and in 1948 the British Medical Association published a report called *The Training of a Doctor*. It was a result of these reports that the Medical Act of 1950 included the requirement of a statutory preregistration year of study in hospital for all medical graduates [see p. 138], and it became generally accepted that medical education did not cease with qualification, but continued throughout life.

In 1957, 100 years after its formation, the General Medical Council issued a set of 'recommendations' which were much less detailed and more permissive than any which had previously been published. These recommendations abandoned the monolithic central control of the details of medical education, and allowed the individual schools a measure of freedom to experiment with teaching, and, to a more limited extent, with the material taught and with the qualifying examinations. Many schools had already initiated some experimentation in their curricula, but had been held back by the necessity of adhering to the semblance of conformity. Since 1957, however, almost all the universities of the British Commonwealth have embarked on an intensive period of soul-searching revision of their ideas and practice. It happened to be in 1957 that the University of Western Australia first opened its doors to medical students (Sinclair, 1958; King, 1958), and thus obtained a head start on all other medical schools under the control of the Council. Other new Australian medical schools followed with their own programmes, but it was several years before the existing British schools, with the momentum inevitably imparted by their existing systems, could discuss, agree, and put into operation curricular changes.

It was also in 1957 that the Association for the Study of Medical Education was founded, with the primary objectives of disseminating and storing information about medical education in different places, and of encouraging and conducting research into matters connected with it (Ellis, 1966a). In 1966 the Association undertook the publication of the *British Journal of Medical Education*; until this time the main forum for discussion of medical education had been the *Journal of Medical Education*, published by the Association of American Medical Colleges. The foundation of the British journal is indicative of the great arousal of interest in medical education in the medical schools of the British Commonwealth.

In 1967, 10 years after relaxing its grip on the details of medical education, the General Medical Council issued another set of recommendations which extended, and in some respects amplified, the attitude which it took in 1957. Medical education was said to consist of four periods: a period of premedical studies, a period of basic medical education (including the so-called preclinical, clinical, and preregistration periods of study), a period of vocational training for a particular career in medicine, and continuous education thereafter for all doctors.

The Council indicated its wish to encourage and increase flexibility in the period of basic medical education. The duration of this period was prescribed as 5 academic years (minimum) followed by 1 year of preregistration study, and it was suggested that senior students should be given more responsibility and fewer examinations, particularly in their final year. The Council recommended that 'a system of continuous or progressive assessment' should be established so that due weight could be given to the student's record throughout his course. Unsatisfactory students were to be identified by this system as early as possible. The Council made no specific recommendations on the timing of any given examination, except for the qualifying examination, which is still determined by statute.

The present official position with regard to development of the means of medical education is thus one of considerable latitude, and the trends of experiment appear to have been welcomed.

DEVELOPMENTS IN THE UNITED STATES

Many, if not all, of the educational ideas current in British and Commonwealth medical schools originally emanated from America, and it is perhaps desirable to include here a brief account of the way in which American medical education developed, in order to explain how experimental curricula could become established there long before this was possible elsewhere in the English-speaking world.

The evolution of medical education in the United States differed considerably from the same process in Britain. There was no unifying General Medical Council, and until early in the twentieth century there was no way of ensuring an adequate and uniform standard of performance from the graduates of the various medical schools, some attached to universities but others purely proprietary, which had grown up in the different States of the Union (Fulton, 1953; Moll, 1968). Standardization of these schools followed the critical report made by Abraham Flexner in 1910 to the Carnegie Foundation for the Advancement of Teaching. This report, the main landmark in American medical education, instituted many reforms, and carried others which had been started to their conclusion, so that many of the inefficient university schools and all the proprietary ones had to close their doors.

Following the report, medical training became a system of 4 years of high school, 4 years of college, and 4 years of medical school (exceptional students might be admitted to a medical school after only 3 years at college). American medical schools instituted a means of voluntary self-regulation in 1906, and nowadays each school is visited every 3 years by teams of 'inspectors' from the joint Liaison Committee on Medical Education of the Association of American Medical Colleges and the American Medical Association (Darley, 1965).

One of the chief educational weapons for ensuring reform was the examination system. In the early days, the examinations conducted by the medical schools for the award of their own diplomas were something of a farce (Moll, 1968), and were completely unsupervised by outside authorities. However, by 1900, 26 of the States had introduced outside examinations, upon which depended the issue of a licence to practise in that State. This system worked well so long as the candidate did not wish to move around from one place to another, but those who did found themselves handicapped, and some sort of agreement between the different States regarding mutual recognition was therefore necessary. Such arrangements grew up piecemeal, and graduates of the institutions in one State might or might not be recognized by all or by a number of the remaining States. It was to counter the uncertainties and difficulties resulting from this situation that the National Board examinations came into being; a graduate who had passed this externally set and assessed examination was recognized as fit to practise by all States in the Union.

The award of a licence thus did not necessarily involve the following of an approved curriculum, but merely the passing of an approved examination—either the State Board or the National Board examinations—and the curricula in different schools could vary considerably. For this reason the dissatisfaction with the orthodox system, which in America, as in Britain, reached its height about the middle of the century, could be translated into action there considerably earlier than it could in Britain. Just after 1945 new methods and new programmes were instituted in many American medical schools (Berry, 1953), the most important of which, because of the heavy impact it made on educational theories, was the programme of the medical school of Western Reserve University [see p. 81].

THE ORTHODOX BRITISH CURRICULUM IN 1957

In 1957 the general shape of the curriculum in British medical schools was still not very different from that which it had assumed in the early years of the century. The details had changed, but the principle was the same.

The time spent by the student was divided horizontally into three

stages. He proceeded from his premedical studies through a preclinical phase to the phase of clinical instruction in the hospital. In
all three phases there was departmental teaching of 'subjects' by
specialists, often without relation to what was being taught in other
specialist departments.

The premedical part of the curriculum might be taken before entry
to the medical school, as in many English schools, or it might form
an integral part of the university curriculum, as in Scotland. In either
case it consisted of a study of physics, chemistry, biology, and
possibly of other subjects, such as genetics.

The preclinical phase of study, always taken at the university, consisted of anatomy, physiology, biochemistry, and pharmacology,
together with other subjects, such as biophysics and statistics, which
varied in extent and in importance from one school to another
(Sinclair, 1955). Pathology and bacteriology, the so-called 'paraclinical' subjects, formed a link between the preclinical and the
clinical teaching.

The clinical part of the curriculum, associated with hospital work,
occupied the last part of the student's instruction, and varied in the
proportions of didactic teaching and clinical experience afforded.
The major clinical subjects were medicine, surgery, obstetrics and
gynaecology, and in some schools paediatrics and psychiatry.

Each 'subject' was examined as the student 'completed' his 'course'
in it, as a necessary prerequisite for proceeding to the next group of
subjects. Each department felt it desirable to give the student as
wide and as good a grounding in its own particular speciality as
possible, probably with the subconscious feeling that this would
increase the prestige and respect for this speciality among the graduates at large. Accordingly, the time available to each department
tended to be fully occupied, and as the subject expanded in scope
and esteem, so the amount of factual material taught to the students
increased.

Much preclinical teaching was done by lectures, and the practical
classes in this period tended to be stereotyped, and to aim at reproducing classical experiments. In the clinical period, lectures were
again prominent, and students were attached to specified wards for
their practical work, being taught by the clinicians on the patients
who happened to be in the ward at the time of attachment.

Examinations were grouped into 'professional' clusters, perhaps
the most formidable being the 'second professional', which occurred
at the end of the preclinical period, and involved anatomy, physiology, and biochemistry, and in some schools pharmacology as well.

The 'final' examinations invariably included medicine, surgery, and midwifery, all examined as separate subjects, and sometimes there were questions on subjects, such as anatomy or physiology, which had already been passed. The general form of the examinations was fairly standard; the questions in the written paper were usually of the essay variety, and in the practical and oral examinations in the preclinical phase the student faced two or more assessors, one of whom was usually an 'external' examiner from another institution. There was a similar arrangement in the clinical examinations, in which the candidate was assessed on his capacity to deal with patients, who were often brought in specially for the purpose because they exhibited certain signs or symptoms.

In the preclinical part of this general system the teachers had to impart the language of medicine, and often the language of English as well. They had to teach students different habits of thought—to wean them away from the parroting of texts and teachers and to bring them nearer the beginnings of independent judgement [see p. 24]. They had to teach the professional aspects of their own particular disciplines—the 'facts' and 'principles' of science in general and of human biology in particular, so that those students passed on to the clinical part of the curriculum would have sufficient understanding, methodology, and vocabulary to benefit from their clinical studies.

The preclinical teachers also had to teach good habits of work, and to stimulate the spirit of inquiry. They had to encourage a scientific attitude towards medical and social problems, many of which might have previously been thought of by their charges only in an emotional context. Finally, they had to detect and exclude unsatisfactory students as quickly as possible, so that they would not place an unnecessary financial burden on the school, and so that their places could be taken by other students more capable of benefiting from the medical course.

The clinicians had an equally onerous responsibility. They had to maintain the scientific approach towards medicine, but to modify it by humanity. They had to impart clinical skills such as history taking, examination, diagnosis, treatment and prognosis, to set a good example in dealing with patients in a considerate and understanding fashion, and finally to bring the student to an understanding of his own limitations as well as his own powers, to advise him on his future career, and to help him with the first steps towards obtaining the necessary grounding for it.

CRITICS AND REFORMERS

Such a system in the past produced many great clinicians and medical scientists. Nevertheless, it engendered serious criticisms, which until recently came from senior members of the profession, mostly clinicians: it was from this quarter that the General Medical Council was influenced when it decided to liberalize its attitude to the curriculum. Following this decision, the ranks of the critics were reinforced by more junior members of the teaching staff, both preclinical and clinical, who brought fresh minds and fresh ideas to bear. This influx was due to an arousal of interest in medical education, stimulated by the possibility of introducing local changes without having to convince a central authority. Each medical faculty nowadays contains a number of reformers who are seeking to build a local pattern to their own specifications, perhaps with the unexpressed idea that such a pattern might provide a standard of excellence copied throughout the English-speaking world. The difficulty is that every such reformer has his own individual 'pet' programme, and often finds it difficult to agree with his colleagues.

Student criticism of medical education is probably as old as medical education itself; for centuries there have been rumblings of discontent, and occasional eruptions into action. But since 1957 there has been a considerable upsurge of interest among students in the methods by which they are converted from raw recruits into medical graduates, and student opinion in most medical schools finds expression in the curriculum committees or in the medical faculty meetings. On a larger scale, the British Medical Students' Association has conducted surveys and made valuable reports on medical education.

Several factors influence the process by which a student entering a medical school evolves into a practitioner of medicine, and some of them are outside the direct control of the medical school—his maturation, his personal contacts, his family problems, his social activities and intellectual interests. But three main factors can be controlled directly. The first of these is the quality of the students, since there are more applicants than places, and selection is universally practised. Theoretically, therefore, the average ability of those accepted, and their enthusiasm and willingness to learn, could be improved by better selection methods. A great deal of work has been put into the problem of selecting students, and immensely complicated systems have been, and are being, used in some medical schools. However, the difficulty of assessing the results of these procedures makes it impossible to say whether or not they are superior to the simpler method of selecting solely on academic achievement (Sinclair, 1955).

The second factor is the quality of the teaching staff, which might be improved by altering the criteria and methods adopted by the selection committees which appoint them. Virtually nothing has been done about choosing teaching staff on the basis of their ability to teach, and this would probably be even more difficult than selecting students.

It is not surprising, therefore, that most of the constructive criticisms of British medical education have been directed against the third main factor directly controlled by the medical schools—the curriculum. Nevertheless, this is rather like treating the symptoms of a disease without attempting to strike at the cause. The curriculum is only a framework, and if the teachers and students are good the products of the school will also be good, for methods are secondary. The success or failure of a school depends not on the timetables, the new teaching methods, or the experimental examinations, but on the people it attracts to teach and study. Nevertheless, in our present state of ignorance it is understandable that we should attempt to tinker with something we think we can control instead of launching out into the unknown, and certainly the orthodox British curriculum in 1957 was open to several objections (Ellis, 1956a).

Perhaps the most insistent of these was that the amount of material taught to the students was constantly growing, stifling their education by the accretion of 'facts' and the accumulation of technological information [see p. 70]. There was very little time left for the student to make up his own mind and form his own opinions on any subject. Coupled with this was the feeling that the time devoted to certain 'subjects' was excessive, and that others received too little attention [see p. 74].

More basic was the criticism that the whole system of uncontrolled departmental teaching led to repetition, disjointed presentation, and disagreement. It was felt that there was a loss of impetus in the early years of the curriculum due to the premedical–preclinical–clinical sequence; students were discouraged at having to embark on a further period of 'basic science' before seeing the relevance of this material and before confronting the sick people they wished to help [see p. 81]. In the preclinical phase students could be excluded from the course purely on the basis of lack of scientific ability, without having had the opportunity of demonstrating their potential as doctors [see p. 143]. Others held that there was too little opportunity for individuality in the curriculum; everyone had to go through the same course irrespective of whether or not it was relevant to his choice of career [see p. 74].

It was claimed that the practical classes left no room for initiative, and that lectures, which dominated the teaching process in most curricula, were not the best means of transferring information and stimulating thought [see p. 102]. At the same time the examination system came in for attack; it was universally agreed that it imposed too heavy a burden, and some maintained that the essay type examination gave an unfair advantage to those who were fluent in English expression [see p. 149].

The last of the major criticisms was that the medical student became isolated from students in other faculties by reason of the amount of supervised work he had to do and because he had to do it in institutions often separated from the university by a considerable distance [see p. 60].

A few of these criticisms were indigenous, but the majority had already been subjected to considerable discussion in the United States and elsewhere [see pp. 9, 11]. Most of them were supported, in this country, by a considerable body of opinion drawn from staff, students, and graduates; others had less widely based encouragement. All of them were value judgements unsupported by any scientific inquiry, and some of them were a trifle overdrawn.[2]

For example, Pickering (1958), one of the severest critics of the orthodox system, claims that medical students suffer through being instructed instead of educated. He contrasts the process of education, in which the student is set to work in his own time, attending lectures 'for not more than two hours a day', and in which the function of the teacher is to appraise his efforts, cure him of bad mental habits, and encourage him in good ones, with the process of instruction, in which nothing is required of the student except to memorize and to reproduce what he remembers. He draws the conclusion that medical education should aim at using the methods of education rather than instruction, and that the teachers should, following Karl Pearson, attempt to impart 'an appreciation of method rather than a knowledge of facts'.

There is considerable force in this argument, but matters are not quite so simple as Pickering makes them. Training for a profession is not the same thing as obtaining a general cultural education, and the idyllic picture he paints of education simply cannot be transferred in its entirety from the arts faculty to the faculty of medicine [see p. 70].

[2] As Fanny Burney said, '. . . the freedom with which Dr. Johnson condemns whatever he disapproves is astonishing'.

Nor can he be whole-heartedly supported when he goes on (Pickering, 1969) to paint a fearsome picture of the evils of medical education before the Medical Act of 1950. He describes departmental teaching as reducing many students to 'intellectual skeletons', and claims that their education 'killed curiosity and initiative'. As Allen (1969) asked with some pertinence, if this is so then how is it that we are still exercising both initiative and curiosity today—or perhaps it is only those who qualified after the Act of 1950 who are doing so? *Are* we all so bad as the reformers would have us believe?

It is perhaps true that only by exaggeration can we be roused to examine our concepts of how things should be done, but the reformers do tend, like the Fat Boy, to make our flesh creep. We hear nothing but ill of the orthodox curriculum, just as we hear nothing but ill of the public school system, for it seems to be only those who were unhappy in both situations who are impelled to write down their feelings; the satisfied customers usually keep silence. Many eminent medical men (including Pickering himself) were dragged through the educational mire which the reformers describe and still survived to lead the profession.

The latest proposals designed to overcome the real or fancied drawbacks of the existing curriculum are those of the Royal Commission on Medical Education, published in 1968. The report of this Commission is a document with which every medical teacher in Britain has had to become familiar, for in most medical schools it has been the subject of extended discussion ever since its publication. The terms of reference of the Commission were 'to review medical education, undergraduate and postgraduate, in Great Britain, and in the light of national needs and resources, including technical assistance overseas, to advise her Majesty's Government on what principles future development . . . should be based . . . to consider what changes may be needed in the pattern, number, nature, or location of the institutions providing medical education or in its general content'. This was a wide brief, and only a relatively small part of the report deals with the undergraduate medical curriculum, which is considered in its setting as part of the overall education of a doctor, from secondary school to the grave.

The main proposal made in the report in relation to the undergraduate curriculum is the institution of a 3-year preclinical course (in a total curriculum of 5 years). This would have a flexible 'modular' structure in which certain topics would be compulsory for all students, others would be available on a 'limited choice' basis, and still others would be offered as completely free 'options'. This proposal, which would convert British medical education into something very like a well-recognized American pattern, depends upon the provision of an extensive postgraduate training programme for which the Government at present shows no signs of being able to provide financial support [see p. 70]. But the report as a whole contains many ideas which, although not new,[3] have stimulated a good deal of thought, and it has therefore provided a valuable service to medical education. These ideas will be discussed later, as they arise.

Like most reports on medical education, the Todd Report is an idealistic statement, and, as the pages turn, it generates a certain air of unreality, both with regard to the proposals for the curriculum and with regard to the assumptions made about the people involved in it. The dedicated student, working without thought of examinations, stooping over his elective project at midnight, faithful in his attendance, full of initiative and perspicacity, is a rare bird in British medical schools [see p. 30], but his existence in large numbers appears to be assumed. Similarly, there are not so many broad-minded and enterprising teachers, capable of devising stimulating presentations, able to write informed reports on every student, and commanding the talent of switching their minds instantaneously from research to teaching and from teaching to medical care or to the completion of idiotic questionnaires, as the report appears to think. When I read material of this kind myself, I bring to mind a student who recently obtained a mark of 2 per cent in his anatomy paper. When I questioned him about this, it emerged that he would be willing to work harder if he were paid more. Until then, he would be content to operate at his present level.

Curricular reform is indeed a happy hunting ground for idealists, and it would be a great pity if it were not so. But the difficulties begin when the idealistic pronouncements of the committees have to be translated into concrete terms by the front-line troops. We are told the qualities desirable in the scientifically based graduate who is our currently fashionable ideal, but how these qualities are to be trained and strengthened, what exactly the student is to be taught, how he is to be induced to think—these matters are spelled out much less clearly. And when it comes to the details of student selection, the production of detailed schedules and of academic timetables, the setting of examinations—all these and much more are left totally vague. Educators tend to be strong on strategy and weak on tactics.

[3] Some are perhaps older than others. Thus Mekie (1969) points out that the general plan of postgraduate education recommended in the report is a 'faithful if modernized' version of the *Ordinances of the Guild of Barber-Surgeons of London*, dated 1556.

In consequence of this the production of each successive general manifesto leads to a long drawn-out and inconclusive series of arguments in each medical school which receives it, together with a positive cataract of paperwork to slake the thirst of the litter of subcommittees whelped by the local curriculum committee.

Some of the educational principles which are discussed by both national and local committees and commissions have been around for long enough to allow them to become crystallized into slogans, and these are perhaps the ones which require the closest attention. Meetings of local curriculum committees often resound with such slogans, which are repeated parrot-wise, without much thought as to the exact meaning and consequences of what is proposed. It is therefore advisable to try to penetrate beyond the slogans to the principles involved, and to examine these basic concepts in the light of both desirability and practicability.

But before doing this we must examine in some detail the background against which these proposals are made—a background which is often too little considered by the planners. In any scheme of reform it is vital to take into account three main factors: the students who will undergo the new curriculum, the teachers who will administer it, and the medical schools in which it is to have its being.

2 Medical Students

'Tis well enough for a servant to be
bred at a university, but the education
is a little too pedantic for a gentle-
man.

Congreve

PREVIOUS EDUCATIONAL EXPERIENCE

It has been said many times that the central figure in medical education is the medical student, and it should not be necessary to repeat
it once more. But those who discuss teaching methods or curricular
changes often seem to forget how essential it is to take into account
the intellectual and psychological characteristics of those who are
to be taught. For example, there are very considerable differences
between American and British medical students (Sinclair, 1955;
Ellis, 1956c; Kemp, 1968), yet ideas developed during the reform of
medical education in America are sometimes adopted uncritically
in Britain without taking into consideration enormously important
factors such as the relative maturity of the students in the two
situations.

On admission to medical school, the American medical student is
usually 20 or 21 years of age, and has already spent 3 or 4 years at
college studying for a basic science degree. Here he has had the
opportunity of enjoying himself and of taking part in social, sporting,
and cultural affairs. When he goes to medical school, he realizes
that 'the halcyon days are over' (Cohen, Hughes, and Richardson,
1957). In contrast, the British medical student is about 18 years of
age, usually comes straight from his secondary school, and has often
had little experience of undirected study. The schooling of British
students is indeed a vital factor in their progress at the university,
and something must be said about it, even though this involves
following a well-trodden path.

Ideally, three things may be expected from the academic education of an intelligent child. The first is that he should acquire an adequate store of basic information. To be able to communicate freely with other people, he must have a command of spoken and written English sufficient to understand complicated instructions and to make his own meaning absolutely clear. He must also know enough mathematics to look after his affairs and to prevent himself from being swindled. Reading, writing, and arithmetic are still the foundations of education, just as they have been for hundreds of years, and on them can be built various superstructures of specialized knowledge suitable for different trades and professions.

The second expectation is that the child should come to look on the pursuit of knowledge as a rewarding activity, and that he should be encouraged to try to find out more about things which particularly interest him. He should learn how to use a library, how to read round a subject, how to listen intelligently to lectures, how to get the best out of the television set. In short, his curiosity should be stimulated.

The third thing that can be expected—or perhaps I should say hoped for—is that the child should learn to think for himself. In the twentieth century this difficult accomplishment is becoming progressively less common. In an age of deadening uniformity, of mass-produced opinions, it is essential that a child should be taught to read and listen critically, rather than unquestioningly, to evaluate evidence, to form his own personal opinions, to be intellectually independent. This final stage, in which the pupil stands on his own intellectual feet, and the relation between teacher and pupil becomes one between senior and junior colleagues, is almost never reached at school, and seldom even in undergraduate courses at the university.

So much for the ideal: what of the reality?

At present the ratio of teachers to pupils, particularly in the vital early stages of school education, makes individual attention very difficult; it is only in the final year or two that the teacher can get to know his pupils thoroughly and appreciate their individual problems; but by this time it may be too late. The child is usually passed on through a succession of different teachers as he rises in the school, never getting to know any one of them well enough to establish much in the way of mutual confidence. He lacks a sense of continuity —not perhaps in the material he is studying, but in the guidance he is receiving, the human side of affairs. Because of the large numbers in the classes, there is no time to discover the views of every individual on any topic which is being discussed, and it is often only the aggressive and extroverted personalities that obtain a hearing, while their less showy colleagues relax gratefully in obscurity, waiting to be told what to think. Hanging unseen over the teacher's desk, like an invisible sword of Damocles, is the spectre of the examinations for the various Certificates of Education. Where so much depends on 'good results' in these examinations, few teachers venture outside orthodoxy, and some even dictate to the class the opinions they should proffer to the examiners. Such an atmosphere is little calculated to stimulate individual or original thought.

In fact, as Wilfred Trotter pointed out, few teachers, whether at school or at university, are prepared to accept original thought when they encounter it. They will gladly allow a student to think for himself, only so long as his thinking does not run counter to their own beliefs. But unless some encouragement towards individuality and critical thought is given in the later stages of schooling, the comfortable habit of dependence may prove too strong for the student ever to reach the stage of making reasoned judgements for himself.

Wyman (1971), speaking at a symposium on secondary school education for medicine, described a common situation: 'Sixth form pupils . . . are being forced through an academic washing machine . . . the fortunate will only be spun dry, and may have a future—the unfortunate will go on through the wringer and will be wrung dry of all future capacity for independent thought. Fortunately, most of our students are resilient and recover, but it always makes me feel sad to meet someone who has worked so hard to achieve A level grades of a sufficiently high standard to gain university entrance that, having obtained a place, he or she is not able to profit from it.'

Another fatal drawback of the modern school system is the lack of emphasis placed on the *use* of the English language. Orthography, sentence construction, punctuation, grammar—all these are now regarded as trivialities, with the inevitable result that most pupils leave school inadequately prepared to express themselves in their native language. This applies particularly to students who have specialized in science at school, for science teachers seldom bother to check or correct the student's ability to communicate—an ability which is nevertheless vital for his academic success. They seem to think that his powers of expression are not relevant, and that, provided he knows a few formulae, or some of the appropriate jargon, they should not penalize him for something which they consider to be none of their business (Aring, 1958). Nothing could be more mistaken. Communication is just as relevant in science as it is in the arts, and the student who cannot cope with it will ulti- mately fail. To quote J. B. S. Haldane: 'I suspect that the most serious criticism of the Science courses in our universities is not their subject-matter, but the fact that Science students have inadequate training in the use of their native language.' To this may be added the comment of V. H. Mottram: 'No one incapable of the accurate use of language can think.' This is not a specialist matter to be dealt with by those who give the formal classes in English—it is something which must permeate every class, and be insisted upon by every teacher. In this instance we are all our brother's keepers.

Not only are students deficient in the ability to write English, many of them are deficient in the ability to understand what other people have written. Part of this trouble is due to the so-called 'progressive' methods of teaching children to read, uncritically copied from America at a time when the Americans were seeking to correct their mistake in adopting them. These methods have contributed to the production of a generation which finds it difficult, and sometimes distasteful, to read. As Barzun (1959) put it, 'Our current discussion of education in America is thus of peculiar interest, because we, dissatisfied with our handiwork, are seeking to change just at the time when England, France and Germany are courageously starting to repeat our mistakes'.

But it is not only English usage which is badly taught. There is a national shortage of science teachers, for most science graduates appear to find it more rewarding to enter industry or a research career rather than to embark on secondary school teaching. The shortage is perhaps particularly apparent in biology, and many schools are unable to give their pupils a grounding in the elements of this subject. Of those that make the attempt, many provide instruction which is at best second-rate, and at worst actively harmful. Yet many would agree with van Oss (1971) that, 'in an ideal Britain, all secondary education would be based on the twin pillars of English and biology'.

But perhaps worst of all the failings of the British school system is our ludicrous national habit of requiring schoolchildren to make up their minds to specialize in either arts or science at the age of puberty (Pickering, 1971). At this age many immature children, afflicted by the troubles of adolescence, have no idea what they want to do, and to compel them at such a time to sacrifice half of their intellectual world is both arrogant and quite unnecessarily cruel. School education should continue to be as general as possible throughout; specialism and professionalism come later.

DIFFICULTIES AND DISTRACTIONS

These, then, are some of the antecedent factors which determine the intellectual profiles of first-year medical students in Britain and which are responsible for many of the difficulties that the less satisfactory students experience when confronted with the medical curriculum. The commonest fault which the members of this subgroup exhibit is an intellectual and psychological immaturity which renders them absolutely dependent on the factual material obtainable from the textbook and the lecture notes they take from the staff. To ask them to make an effort to find out something for themselves, or to form an opinion of their own from the facts presented, is to ask something quite outside their experience. This criticism may be more applicable to Scottish students than to English ones, who may have had some experience of working on their own in sixth-form study, and are to this extent more mature. One might expect that their difficulties would be solved in the course of the premedical year of the Scottish curriculum, but the sheer size of first-year university classes often renders individual remedial treatment impracticable. As a result, even in the preclinical stage of the curriculum the majority of the class have little idea of how to work, and often come for advice. Because of their dependence upon a steady stream of predigested 'facts' dictated by their teachers, they are lost when the lecturers do not attempt to cover the whole subject, and may also complain bitterly if they go too fast for the students to take down every word. Nor do they question what they are being taught, or consider means whereby it might be verified, for they have little critical faculty, and very few have developed any originality of thought. Some are suspicious of advice given by their teachers, and look on them as potential enemies rather than potential friends. The scars of coaching techniques are obvious on the minds of many of them, and they learn by rote instead of trying to understand what they are taught. Possibly for this reason they are very deficient in observation, and much prefer to recite from the book rather than to direct their attention to what they can see for themselves. They attend only to 'examinable' material, and omit any attempt at collateral reading. Nevertheless, this narrow-mindedness does them little good, for when it comes to the examination we find that they do not know how to arrange their thoughts in logical order, how to select from the mass of data available the things which are relevant and important, or how to use them to construct a meaningful story which is both succinct and readable. In short, they cannot answer the standard sort of essay question with any assurance or competence.

Nor can they follow simple written instructions. In essay type examinations they misread both the general instructions and the questions with an alarming regularity, and answer completely without regard to what was asked. Their thinking is often extremely woolly, and many of them appear to be satisfied with essays which, though they might do credit to a 14-year-old student of nature study, are quite out of place in a university. Some have no idea of how to spell, how to write an ordinary English sentence, how to make themselves clearly understood. There was a time when the structure of an English sentence was recognized for the mighty thing it is, but the memory of these days has long been buried under a welter of phonetic spelling, verbs which do not agree with their subjects, and commas scattered at random throughout the page. Yet the students who write in this way are theoretically the cream of the production of the schools.

As time goes on every medical student matures and grows older, and as he does so, he faces additional hazards. In his first year his time is spent very largely in enjoying the comparative freedom of university life, investigating his capacity for beer, and participating in sport. The second year is employed in furthering his acquaintance with the opposite sex and in going to parties, which often last all night. In the third year twenty-first birthday parties break out and spread like measles. The fourth year sees further extensive investigations among the other sex, which may lead, in the fifth year, to marriage, and in the sixth year to the arrival of a baby (or occasionally vice versa). This routine may lead, in extreme cases, to failure in the course, and the provision of tablets to suppress the libido of medical students might have an incalculable effect on failure rates.

Coupled with these delights, some exhibit an overwhelming desire to participate in student politics, which has been the downfall of many promising entrants. Similar traps are provided by such activities as writing articles for student publications or by an undue enthusiasm for the support of student societies. All these things in themselves are praiseworthy, for they tend to broaden the outlook of the immature student. Nevertheless, with a sad lack of balance, a few indulge in them to such excess that this in itself produces failure.

A similar lack of sense of proportion sometimes bedevils those who play sport. In the old days in London and the ancient universities it was well recognized that many students came up largely to play sport and only secondarily to take part in any academic activity. The pressure of modern life and the expense of education, which

CBE

involves the acceptance of grants from public funds, and necessitates weeding out the class as early as possible, has now rendered this attitude untenable. Yet many medical students, who, along with students of dentistry and engineering, show a tendency towards mesomorphism (Harrison, Weiner, Tanner, and Barnicott, 1964), find the lure of university athleticism of one kind or another irresistible, and risk their academic careers by incessant practice in their desire to represent the university in a more physical capacity. It is traditional to urge every new student to play some regular team sport because of its character-building effects, but each time I see free fights developing during the course of certain team sports I begin to wonder just what *kind* of characters they are building. It is impossible to deny the medical value of regular exercise, but it is equally certain that sport, though a good servant, is an intolerable master.

Finally, there is the question of finance. Nowadays, virtually every student whose family circumstances demand it obtains a grant of some kind to enable him to survive during the period of his education in a British medical school. The way this grant is spent is within the control of the student, who is often, at least in the early stages, not very skilled in managing his money. As a consequence, many students pass from a state of undreamed-of wealth at the time of arrival of their grant to a state of penury towards the end of the session, the process being hastened in many cases by expenditure on beer, cigarettes, cars, and other former luxuries which are nowadays considered absolutely basic necessities. As a result, food may be the subject of economy, and the examinations may be undertaken in poor physical and mental shape.

It is partly for financial reasons that the traditional Australian practice of dropping everything the moment the examinations are over and getting down to the 'real business' of earning one's living in the vacation is spreading in Britain. It is difficult to make students realize that university vacations are not intended either as mere holidays or as opportunities to make money, unless this is absolutely necessary to pay next year's fees and board. I know personally several students who have actually thrown away their chances of getting through supplementary examinations, and thus their future careers, for the sake of making a few pounds of unnecessary pocket money. The idea that vacation work represents 'real life', and that fitting oneself for a profession by reading or obtaining further experience is in some way an inferior activity, has no place in the modern world.

These are general problems. But other stressful situations are provided by the medical course itself (Miller *et al.*, 1961). There is first the fear of failure, of being unable to cope with the course material; this manifests itself chiefly in relation to the numerous examinations which punctuate the curriculum. Every student health service knows well the upsurge of psychosomatic complaints which precede the annual examinations, and which, together with the frank anxiety states and psychiatric disturbances, constitute a major part of their work. A good deal of curious behaviour during the early stages of the course may be traced to this fear of inadequacy; otherwise intelligent students may simply throw in the towel and cease to attend classes or to do any work for fear of subjecting themselves to evaluation and being found wanting.

In the early stages of the curriculum the 'late developers' are still confronting the psychological difficulties of adolescence. Such students may become anxious when transplanted to an unaccustomed environment, and a number of them may develop overt psychiatric states under the stress of the situation. A particularly difficult time is the introduction to the dissecting room; even today death is a solemn subject, hedged around with taboos, and some students are emotionally upset by this experience—a few even to the extent of having to give up the course.

In their third year British medical students are prone to suffer from a number of fancied mortal diseases; those who discover their perfectly normal pelvic colon when practising abdominal palpation in the bath may develop a transient carcinoma of the colon, and those who detect a few extrasystoles may resign themselves to an incurable cardiac condition. Usually these illnesses do not last long, for they clear up spontaneously with the increase of knowledge, but they may be the cause of considerable anxiety for a time.

Some students find the transition from preclinical to clinical work an anxious time, and the first few physical examinations of patients may be disturbing, for the necessity for physical exposure violates much that the student has been taught to believe about modesty and personal privacy. Psychiatry is another testing stage; the student is often brought up sharply against his own emotional difficulties by endeavouring to understand those of other people, and until he has become reconciled to the new insights he gains into behaviour, particularly sexual behaviour and sexual problems, he may go through a very trying period.

Finally, in the later stages of clinical work, many students become upset by having to accept clinical responsibility for the patients under their care.

EFFECTS OF MATURATION AND EDUCATION

As he passes through the medical course, every student has the opportunity of educating himself—the phrase is 'educating himself' rather than 'becoming educated', for the process is an active and not a passive one. The medical curriculum can provide a most satisfactory education for those who take the trouble to acquire it. Yet for every well-educated medical graduate there are a dozen who are merely well-informed. These are the ones whose capacity for understanding and wisdom has become buried deep beneath the pile of technical information. Factual knowledge, valuable though it is, can only form a basis for an education, not an end in itself, and only those who use the factual details to fertilize rather than to stifle their reasoning powers are able to profit by the intangible factors in the curriculum which convert an accomplished technician into an educated man.

During the slow unfolding of the medical course many qualities can be acquired in addition to the primary one of being able to exercise individual critical thought. At the beginning, the legacy of unsatisfactory secondary education and the abrupt transition from school to university combine to render it difficult for the student to do much more than learn to keep his head above water. Yet throughout the animal kingdom this lesson in self-preservation is the first essential which has to be learned in order to ensure the survival of the species.

Later, the study of anatomy, quite apart from the content of the course, affords the student an opportunity (not always taken; Roberts, 1948; Chance and Humphries, 1966) to observe instead of merely looking, to describe his findings accurately and concisely, and to think logically and consecutively. His memory is trained by stretching it, and at this stage many students find out for the first time how to use their own language with clarity and precision.

Physiology is the foundation for that capacity to argue which is the core of the 'art' as well as the 'science' of medicine. Where so much is uncertain it is essential to acquire the knack of distinguishing the probable from the unlikely, of weighing the evidence and coming to a provisional conclusion which can then be tested. These aptitudes of analysis and synthesis lead on to a capacity for differential diagnosis, and ultimately to the rarest of all human qualities, commonsense. Both physiology and biochemistry inculcate the habit of critical evaluation of every so-called 'fact' presented for consumption, and both induce in the student a way of thought which is applicable to the problems and difficulties of his whole future life. This 'scientific method' is reinforced by the paraclinical disciplines of microbiology and pathology, in which the student learns more deeply the importance of apparently trivial facts and the value of systematizing his observations. In the clinical years the handling of patients brings—to those whose minds are prepared for it—the quality of humility, coupled with a willingness to accept responsibility in spite of ignorance. The curiosity fostered by preclinical training is now modified by the development of tact and discretion. The ability to select facts and separate out the vital portions of any problem from the incidentals is gradually improved with increasing experience, but just as important is another quality which is also only too rare—imagination. It is this that allows the educated doctor to put himself in the position of his patient, and it is this that brings with it true sympathy and compassion.

At every stage it is the student himself, the individual, who must make the major effort. He whose mind is insufficiently plastic to adapt itself to the changing circumstances of its environment may make a skilled medical tradesman but nothing more. Fortunately there is constantly at hand a means of broadening and developing his outlook, for he has around him, in the class of which he is a member, a group of other people who are going through the same experience. He is not alone. It is one of the tenets of all residential universities that students do a better job of educating each other than is done by the staff.[1] The endless hours of talk, the cups of coffee, the society meetings—all these, if kept in perspective, are potent educational factors and must be treated with respect. The student who retires every night with his books to the seclusion of his room and who denies himself any outside contact because of an anatomy oral test the next week is not educating himself. He may get through his examinations, but he will never be an educated man. It is one of the tragedies of medical education that so many are driven, by the sheer quantity of material to be mastered, to do just this.

An enormous part in the education of medical students is played by the patients upon whom they practise their growing skills, both technical and humanitarian. The lessons they teach are not merely medical ones, and nobody with any sensibility can pass through a medical course without acquiring a sense of wonderment at human

[1] Stephen Leacock, discussing Oxford, said, 'If I were founding a university I would found first a smoking room; then when I had a little more money I would found a dormitory; then after that, or more probably with it, a decent reading room and library. After that, if I still had more money that I couldn't use, I would hire a professor and get some textbooks'.

decency and fortitude, as well as an appreciation of the depths of human depravity and selfishness. Despite the inconvenience of being examined, sometimes by relays of students, patients are usually very well disposed towards them, and many a desperate candidate in the final examination owes his pass to a co-operative and intelligent patient with a soft heart.

Behind the patients stand the nursing staff, who have determined the whole future, domestic as well as professional, of so many doctors. It is extremely educative to be told off in public by an irate ward sister, and not less instructive to drink tea with a glamorous night nurse at 2 a.m. It is perhaps unfortunate that the first of these experiences is so common, while the second is so much the prerogative of the residents as to be exceedingly rare; but both have an incalculable effect on future behaviour.

The medical course exercises its effects not only on education but also on character. The reputation for wildness acquired by medical students in the last century (Dalrymple-Champneys, 1955) still surrounds them like a rather disreputable halo. A hundred years ago the students of St. George's Hospital were, as Sir Henry Acland said, 'the most bearish I have ever beheld as a mass. . . . The whole tone is essentially low-bred'. In those days students used to drink, smoke, and brawl in the dissecting room, and 'distinguished members of the profession would commonly tell utterly indecent and dirty stories in their lectures'. Bob Sawyer and his friends who entertained Mr. Pickwick were in fact no exaggerations, but may even be regarded as underdrawn (Merskey, 1969).

Nowadays things are rather different, but it is still mildly astonishing that a group of students, even now associated in the public mind with wild behaviour and unlicensed horseplay, should suddenly become transformed, by the award of a degree, into the grave and highly polished men of the world we see walking the wards of their teaching hospital in the pride of their first house appointment. The answer is, I think, that the student is throughout his period of education developing like a moth inside a cocoon; the outer shell retains the semblance it had in the earlier stages of its growth, but inside are quietly and imperceptibly growing the qualities and strengths necessary for the tremendous change-over into a new environment. Those of us who are privileged to watch this metamorphosis inevitably find it fascinating. Like the Duke of Plaza-Toro, we lead our regiments from behind, but unlike him we find it more, not less, exciting.

All this adds up to the fact that the medical student who enters the medical course is a very different creature from the one who leaves it in possession of his medical degree. It is true that some have brilliancies of mind and qualities of character which are immediately apparent in the earliest stages, and equally there are others who do not seem to develop intellectually or psychologically despite all their experiences. However, the majority of the class grow up both physically and mentally during the medical course, and innovations in teaching methods or content can often provoke very different reactions according as they are applied early or late in the curriculum.

It is this which makes it extremely inadvisable for British medical schools to use, without due consideration, the methods which have characterized the reform of the American medical curriculum. To ask students with the degree of commonsense, literacy, and enthusiasm typical of the 'tail' of the British class in the early stages of the curriculum to undertake individual experimental work, to allow them to have most of their time free for individual study, to excuse them the necessity for passing any examinations—all this sort of thing is quite out of place in the early years. Later, as in the American curriculum, the students can make a better attempt at dealing with such situations.

George Miller, accustomed to American students, has said that students ought to be treated like scholars, not like schoolboys, for only in this way will they learn to behave like scholars; he cites Bernard Shaw's opinion that 'a lady is a lady because she is treated like a lady'. But in the earliest part of the British curriculum the student *is*, in all essentials, a schoolboy, and it is futile to expect him to behave otherwise until he has grown up a little. The transition from schoolboy to scholar spans the duration of the curriculum, and the difference between the callow youth of the first year and the staid and responsible married man in the final year is too great to be ignored in any scheme of medical education.

STUDENT NUMBERS

In Britain, medicine no longer attracts those applicants with the very best academic qualifications; this may be because of the length, expense, and supposed difficulty of the course, because of the poor public image of the National Health Service, or because of the attractions of novel careers such as nuclear physics or computer technology. The average intelligence quotient of medical students has in the past tended to be lower than those of students in the faculties of arts or science (Eysenck, 1953). Although every medical student has satisfied the entrance requirements of the university, these are always *minimal* requirements,[2] and are usually set fairly low so as to avoid penalizing good students who for some reason may not have been able to reach a high standard at school. The student body in the early stages of the medical course may thus exhibit a very considerable range of academic ability, from the excellent at one end to the completely unsuitable at the other.

Currently, the medical schools in Britain are being urged to take in ever increasing numbers of medical students, and the inescapable conclusion is that these additional numbers will be drawn from people even less able to cope with the medical course than those at the bottom of the present classes. Although far more students still apply for medicine than the universities can accommodate, many of the applicants are of poor quality, and the total number of applicants may be decreasing, though information on this point is difficult to obtain. Selection methods (Sinclair, 1956a) are probably inaccurate when they try to take account of factors other than academic ability, and most schools rely fairly heavily on demonstrated performance in the examinations for the Certificates of Education (Perry, 1966). Yet even this does not correlate as well as might be expected with performance in the medical course.

The cry of the time is for quantity rather than quality, and an increase in intake may in itself determine a change in educational methods. A class of 80 can be taught in ways very different (and usually much more satisfying to both teachers and taught) from the methods applicable to a class of 160. This is particularly the case if the extra students come (as they must do if our selection methods mean anything at all) from a group with lower intellectual levels than the others. When the expansion has taken place, classes will have a much longer 'tail' than they do at present, and failure rates will undoubtedly go up if present standards are maintained.

The danger is that the need of the country for doctors will so impress those concerned with medical education that imperceptibly the standard will be lowered, so that the failure rate remains fairly steady. For some years some educationists have been maintaining that 'more' does not necessarily mean 'worse' while others have maintained that deterioration is inescapable. It is a measure of the pitiable uncertainties which surround education as a whole that the protagonists of both sides of the argument rest their case largely on

[2] Jones, R. V., *Times Educational Supplement*, 27 February 1970.

simple affirmation, for irrefutable evidence is incredibly difficult to muster. Nevertheless, it seems unarguable that if additional staff are not provided to deal with the extra numbers (and this seems very likely in view of the current difficulties in obtaining staff) the addition of a large number of academically weak students to the class must inevitably produce disabilities. In large classes it is not only those towards the bottom who suffer; the bright students receive less individual attention, and are deprived of the stimulation which this attention may bring with it. We may expect a reduction in the achievement of those at the top as well as a deterioration in performance of those at the bottom.

It is sad to think that this will be received with perfect equanimity by both educationists and Government alike. The concept of 'quality' in education is on its way out, and the only criterion nowadays is that of expense. The dominance of money in all matters educational has led to the concept of 'productivity' (Blaug, 1968), which in essence means: how many cattle can be herded through the stockade in the minimum time, to emerge, groggily, with their certificate of attendance branded on their flanks? It appears inevitable that God is to be on the side of the big battalions, and that classes will increase in size until somebody decides that too many doctors, not too few, are being produced, when they will swing back again to a figure which will probably prove to be much too low. The criterion determining this up and down sine curve of production, which has been going on since the last war, is largely an economic one. The situation is complicated by the decision of many of the better students, often early in their course, to emigrate on qualification. This decision is based not only on financial grounds; it may arise in part from a wish to see the world and to take part in the affairs of a young energetic growing country, or from an impatience with the often stultifying bureaucratic pressures of the National Health Service. One cannot blame intelligent students with initiative for wishing to make the best use of these qualities, but it is a pity that much of the cream of the class disappears while the skimmed milk remains.[3]

Conversely, the number of overseas students in British medical schools is decreasing, largely because of the very considerable increase in fees inflicted on such students some years ago. On the whole they were keen and enthusiastic, and often better prepared to work hard

[3] Last (1968) considers that the Royal Commission on Medical Education took too pessimistic a view of the future drain of emigration. He believes that if conditions in Britain were to improve, far fewer doctors would emigrate. Nevertheless, the problem is currently a big one. Gish (1970) estimates that in the 5 years 1962–67 approximately 400 British trained doctors emigrated each year in excess of those who returned.

than British students of the less satisfactory kind; they were therefore in many ways a good influence.

One of the worst aspects of the increase in numbers in the medical schools of this country, and, indeed of the increase of numbers in other faculties also, is the resultant expansion of administrative services largely unconnected with teaching and learning. The innumerable committees and the proliferation of paperwork inevitably require the attention of staff who would otherwise be engaged in the more productive and rewarding work of teaching and research [see p. 49]. Already in 1934 Sir Henry Tizard thought that the universities were too full to have an atmosphere in which learning, individuality, and self-reliance could flourish. The tendency of numbers, he thought, was towards over-organization, too little latitude, and too much spoon-feeding. 'The wider we fling open the doors to a university, the more will such organization be necessary, and the worse will be the conditions for the best teachers and students.'

Medical classes in this country have not yet reached the size of some of those in the faculties of arts and science, where a single department may have to cater for more than 1000 students within its walls.[4] Under such conditions it is very difficult for a student to feel any sense of individuality, and the inevitability of being treated as an administrative unit rather than as a person diminishes his sense of confidence and increases his sense of futility. It is surely no accident that the bulk of student unrest in this country has its roots in the faculties of arts and social sciences, where many students with too little to do in the way of supervised work are herded together in enormous classes and have no clear indication of how their future lives are to be spent. The students in the medical faculty, who have the advantage of a well-defined objective and a readily expressed set of ideals, are so far less prone to excesses in the direction of student 'protest' than their colleagues. Few medical deans have as yet been tied up in their offices to allow the infuriated student body to ransack the files for political evidence. Nevertheless, a small minority of medical students are already much more interested in their 'rights' than in learning, and the number may be expected to increase as the classes swell.

Concurrent with this is the great increase in the amount of committee participation which it is nowadays fashionable to ask the students to undertake. Most medical schools have staff/student committees—sometimes in each department—and students often sit

[4] But in the University of Sydney 650 medical students began first-year medicine in 1963.

as observers at faculty meetings. This consultation of student opinion can be very valuable in relation to matters such as curricular innovations, but it has to be remembered that students who *get* on to committees are usually students who are *anxious* to get on to committees; it is a truism that student representatives are rarely representative students.

Exactly how much attention should be paid to student views on teaching and content of the curriculum is doubtful. As Ashby and Anderson (1970) point out, if doctors and professors do not know more than patients and students, there is no point in having hospitals and universities at all. Yet the only expertise of doctor or professor which patient or student is obliged to acknowledge is the expertise which brings the two together; outside this no authority can be claimed. The problem is, therefore, how to define the margins of this 'expertise'. Students are, rightly, apt to complain if they do not see and understand the rationale of any new development, and a great many difficulties can be avoided if machinery for the swift communication and explanation of new proposals to the student body exists; nothing is more vital to the success of educational planning. But student opinion as to the necessity for this or that in the medical course naturally carries less weight than the opinions of those who have already seen the curriculum as a whole and who know what lies beyond it.

STUDENT PSYCHOLOGY

Medical students form a very diverse group, and, in spite of innumerable questionnaires designed to establish their motivation and psychological characteristics, all that can be said is that these characteristics cannot be specified with any certainty.

Some medical students embark on a medical career through a sense of idealism, in the desire to help humanity. Such people often become discouraged by the early stages of the curriculum, which may seem to them very far removed from healing the sick. This is perhaps particularly the case in Scotland, where the first year of the curriculum repeats a good deal of school work for the benefit of those students who did not have the opportunity of covering this material at school. As a result, between 40 and 50 per cent of them are assailed by doubts regarding their choice of career (Brotherston, Martin, and Boddy, 1963). As time goes on, the initial idealism becomes converted, in many cases, to a superficial and probably protective cynicism; so much so that the preclinical and clinical phases of the curriculum are sometimes spoken of as the precynical and the cynical phases of medical education (Becker and Geer, 1958b).

Other students have been nudged into their present surroundings by family pressure, or by the prospect of a reasonably paid and secure job. As a result they may have little interest in medicine for its own sake, and are frequently completely ignorant of matters pertaining to their chosen profession. If I ask them about Louis Pasteur or Lord Lister, I meet with blank incomprehension, and I am sure that similar stories could be told by most other teachers in the faculty of medicine. It is, of course, axiomatic that all students in danger of being ejected from the medical school because of unsatisfactory performance are devoted to medicine and have never for a moment considered any other career. This tendency is particularly strong in those who have failed to attend classes or who have obtained less than 15 per cent in their annual examinations. It is also axiomatic that many such students have, during their course, suffered some powerful personal anxiety which has completely interfered with their normal standard of achievement.

In Britain, doctoring runs in the family; about 20 per cent of the students questioned in the ASME survey were the sons or daughters of doctors.[5] But with the vast expansion of tertiary education in all English-speaking countries, an increasing proportion of medical students is drawn, not only from non-medical families, but from families with no previous experience of university education of any kind. Some of these families have little sympathy with, and may even exhibit contempt for, the rigorous training of mind which is necessary. The student may thus find himself without any backing for his ambitions and ideals in his home surroundings, and the conflict set up by this situation may act deleteriously on his work.

The newcomers from non-medical families often have very little idea of what they will have to do in their medical course, and their concept of medicine is very vague. Some think it is a great body of known facts (Ellis, 1956c; Becker and Geer, 1958a) which has to be mastered, and when it becomes obvious that they cannot learn everything, they worry about what is 'important'. Indeed, they form their own concepts of this, and, despite the efforts of their teachers, they may fail to learn such matters as the blood supply of the heart 'because I didn't think it was important'. Conversely, they may set

[5] Report of the Royal Commission on Medical Education, 1968.

themselves some enormous and unproductive task, such as learning in detail the ossification of the skull, because for some reason one of their colleagues thought this was a certain 'spot' for the examination. It is one of the more consistent characteristics of medical students as a group (as it is of humanity at large) that they are credulous of what is told them by anyone other than those who are paid to do the telling.

The very spread of tertiary education has led to a lessening of the respect for it. University education was formerly thought to be a valuable thing in itself; nowadays it is increasingly regarded as a course of training leading to a degree, which in turn provides a meal ticket. This attitude, common among both families and students, means that the object of most students is simply to pass the examinations which bar their way. It is extremely difficult to convince them that they ought to be acquiring habits of thought which they will need in their professional lives; they want merely to 'get through' each subject as they come to it. The old and laudable idea that it is as well to do one's best in any circumstances is now out of fashion, and is being supplanted by the belief that it is sufficient to get $49\frac{1}{2}$ per cent and be pushed through the turnstile with the mob.

Some students are 'convergers' by nature, enjoying logical and well-defined arguments, liking to know where they stand, and whether they are 'right' or 'wrong'; they prefer technical to personal or emotional matters. In contrast are the 'divergers', who enjoy uncertainty and prefer argument to logical or technical material. There is some evidence that convergers and divergers may each prefer to be taught by similarly-minded teachers (Joyce and Hudson, 1968).

Nowadays many medical students are women (the figures in 1966–67 varied from 11 per cent to 50 per cent in different British schools), but little attention has been paid to the possible differences between the ability of male and female students to cope with or to benefit from the medical course. Walton (1968) has reported that women in their fifth year of the Edinburgh curriculum were found to be more competent than men, as well as being more able students; they were also more introverted than the men, and more anxious, but less prone to feel that their teachers gave them insufficient guidance, and better prepared to take responsibility.

A study of graduating medical students in the same school revealed four kinds of doctor, based on the grouping of certain attributes (Walton, Drewery, and Phillip, 1964). Combining these attributes to form a composite picture, two of the type specimens were oriented towards organic illness, and two were interested in social and emotional aspects of illness. Of the first pair, one was considered to be 'adequate' in his attitudes, and the other 'limited'; this one was impatient with those who do not have serious organic illness. Of the last pair, one was 'research-oriented', and the other was 'patient-centred', suggesting a possible career as a psychiatrist.

It is of course very desirable that there should be diverse types of personality among the students, for no profession can offer a greater variety of jobs to its entrants. Nevertheless this lack of uniformity means that it is difficult to frame a curriculum which will satisfy everybody. From this basic fact spring some of the tremendous variety of criticisms to which the orthodox curriculum has been subjected, and also the desire to 'personalize' the medical course [see p. 94].

3 Teachers

'Sound scholar' is a term of praise
applied to one another by learned
men who have no reputation outside
the University...A lecturer is a sound
scholar, who is chosen to teach on
the ground that he was once able to
learn.
Francis Cornford,
Microcosmographia Academica

RECRUITMENT

The person who has most chance to influence the thinking of the
next generation is the school teacher, who is thus one of the most
important people in the community. By the time a boy gets to the
university, his thinking patterns are well established, and in many
cases it is too late for university teachers to do much about improving them. The future of medical education thus depends basically
on what goes on at school, and it could even be said that the most
important figure in medical education is the primary school teacher.

If a schoolboy or a university student is intelligent and enthusiastic,
he will survive a great deal of bad teaching. But if, like the majority,
he has difficulties both with the subject matter and with the methods
of study, the help and stimulation provided by a good teacher is of
inestimable value, and the lack of them may mean the difference
between success and failure.

The teacher has been described as an enzyme: on one side of him
is the subject matter to be digested, and on the other the student
who has to absorb it. In the last century such 'enzymes' were highly
regarded for their abilities, both by students, colleagues, and the
general public (Sinclair, 1955). It was in this phase that Nietzsche
remarked to Burckhardt that he 'would very much prefer a professorial chair in Basle to being God'. Even up to the beginning of the
Second World War the teacher, both in school and in university,

was a respected figure. University teachers were indeed expected by this time to do some research, but the assessment of their worth did not depend exclusively on this side of their activities, and their capacity as teachers was alone sufficient to ensure them a place in public esteem. But since 1945 the idea has become current that it is more praiseworthy to find out new facts or formulate new theories than it is to guide the minds of the young. Practising teachers, like practising doctors, have lost a great deal of the respect that they were formerly accorded, and are now almost universally thought to be less valuable to the community than research workers. As Barzun has said, 'Teaching is not a lost art, but the regard for it is a lost tradition'. As a result, selection for senior academic posts now depends very largely on the number and quality of the research publications submitted,[1] and teaching ability or organizational capacity is relegated to a position of subordinate importance. Recently, with the emergence of interest in medical education, it has become mandatory for selection committees to ask a few questions about the candidate's views on the reform of the curriculum, but his ability to teach is still not explored in any way.

The attitude that research is more important than teaching is shared by many of the teachers themselves, who would really prefer to work in a research institute, and take on a teaching post only as a method of obtaining research facilities. Their dreams are not of turning out impeccably educated graduates, but of Nobel Prizes, knighthoods, Fellowships of the Royal Society, and so on. Such people may eventually be appointed to senior teaching posts without ever having acquired more than a nodding acquaintance with the parts of their subject which lie outside the scope of their own research interests. The situation was well described by Richard de Bury in 1345: 'But, painful to relate, the clerks who are famous in these days pursue a very different course [from the ancients]. Afflicted with ambition in their tender years, and slightly fastening to their untried arms the Icarian wings of presumption, they prematurely snatch the master's cap; and mere boys become unworthy professors

---

[1] This is one of the facts of life which all medical teachers have to contend with, and it leads to a great deal of unnecessary research of poor quality. Platt (1967), talking about clinical research, points out that 'given a new and expensive tool such as a gas chromatograph, an electromagnetic flowmeter, or a multichannel recorder of some kind, it becomes all too easy to find a subject for research; for there is bound to be something which has not yet been measured by these means. The need for thought, observation, ideas, and hypothesis, which form the hard work of research, recedes comfortably into the background for a year or two, while the research worker, supported by a grant and relieved of the much harder task of practising medicine, collects his results and has them analysed for him by a computer'.

of the several faculties, through which they do not make their way step by step, but like goats ascend by leaps and bounds; and having slightly tasted of the mighty stream, they think that they have drunk it dry, though their throats are hardly moistened. And because they are not grounded in the first rudiments at the fitting time, they build a tottering edifice on unstable foundations, and now that they have grown up, they are ashamed to learn what they ought to have learned while young, and thus they are compelled to suffer for ever for too hastily jumping at dignities they have not deserved.'

The general view is that research provides an excitement which is lacking in teaching, but, like so many general views, it is mistaken. Routine research work is just as dull and tedious as routine teaching, and the moments of excitement are few and far between. Nor are they all on one side of the balance. A good example of the excitement of teaching, which I personally find rather moving, occurs in the film *My Fair Lady* when Eliza Doolittle succeeds in mastering the sentence: 'The rain in Spain stays mainly on the plain'. This moment seems to me to epitomize the attraction of teaching. The careful preparation, the attention to detail, the co-operation with the pupil to a common end, and, finally, the joint creation of something that did not exist before—a skill, a habit of thought, the understanding of a difficult problem—this provides a satisfaction at least equal to that of recording and compiling the responses of a rabbit to a new drug, or that of investigating the blood chemistry of 1000 consecutive patients with some chronic metabolic disorder.

For the dedicated teacher, such delights may well be enough, and many teachers in the past have been willing to labour under the most unsatisfactory conditions, both as regards accommodation and equipment. But this is a financially-minded century, in which materialism is prone to overwhelm such idealism as most people can muster. In many of the professions in which the 'call to duty' was formerly sufficient to ensure recruitment, salary and conditions of work are now becoming the leading factors in attracting new entries. This again is not a new situation, and Francis Bacon spoke of 'the defect which is in public lectures; namely, in the smallness and meanness of the salary or reward which in most places is assigned to them. . . . For it is necessary to the progession of sciences that Readers be of the most able and sufficient men. . . . This cannot be, except their condition and endowment be such as may content the ablest man to appropriate his whole labour . . . in that function and attendance.' The teaching profession as a whole has too long had inadequate financial compensation and is now in revolt.

DBE

The specialized teachers who work in the preclinical departments of the medical schools have less to complain of in an absolute sense, but the medically qualified preclinical teacher is at a very considerable disadvantage compared to those of equal ability who happen to have chosen to take up clinical work. In the preclinical departments at Aberdeen the salaries for the career post of senior lecturer are at present 28 per cent below the comparable clinical salaries at the bottom of the scale and 44 per cent below them at the top of the scale (Kelman, 1971). Elsewhere, the situation is similar, and it has been estimated that the overall career earnings of a clinical senior lecturer are likely to be at least £50,000 in excess of those of his preclinical counterpart (Martin *et al.*, 1971). Appointment to a preclinical chair usually takes place at about the age of 45, whereas appointment to National Health Service consultant status usually occurs at about the age of 35; there is no progressive salary scale for preclinical professors such as obtains for consultants. Not only is this so, but consultants (and senior full-time clinical teaching staff) also have the opportunity of obtaining a distinction award in the National Health Service. The maximum (salary plus award) a clinical professor can hope to reach is currently considerably more than double the maximum for a preclinical medically qualified professor. Though few clinicians receive a maximum award, most have a substantial supplementation under the scheme, and, even taking into account the inroads of taxation, a strong financial incentive is provided to take up clinical rather than preclinical work (Davidson, 1971).

The argument for paying clinical teachers more is that their work entails the care of patients, and this would at once be accepted by most preclinical teachers as a justification for a differential. However, many medical graduates receive clinical salaries although they have no routine National Health Service commitment and may never see a patient. As Hill (1971) put it, 'Higher clinical salaries are justified on the grounds of giving extra payment for "clinical responsibility"; yet with the increasing infiltration of academic clinical departments by experimentalists and medical scientists, as well as the proliferation of paraclinical departments (who share the cornucopia), the argument now seems hardly tenable'. Conversely, many medically qualified preclinical teachers take part, without additional remuneration, in the training and examination of medical postgraduates and in the work of clinical units.

An established teacher devoted to a preclinical subject may accept such differentials with no more than moderate resentment—after all, he has no clinical worries, he is not called out of bed at night, and his teaching year, though sometimes longer than that of his colleagues in other scientific disciplines, is usually considerably shorter than that of a clinical teacher. But for those who are hesitating about whether to choose a preclinical or a clinical career, the financial disability is usually decisive, and fewer and fewer medical graduates are being recruited into the preclinical departments. For example, from 1950 to 1960 the percentage of medically qualified staff in British departments of physiology was fairly constant at about 66 per cent, but by 1970 the figure had declined to 48 per cent, the decline being particularly rapid in the last 5 years. Of the remaining medically qualified staff, over 30 per cent were due to retire within the 10 years following 1970. In 1965, four out of five applicants for vacant teaching posts in physiology were medically qualified, but in 1970 the proportion was one in five, and fewer were being appointed.

Not only are there fewer recruits, but more and more medically qualified staff already in posts are leaving after a short stay to join the ranks of the clinicians. The situation is also aggravated by the advent of new medical schools, which compete with each other for medically qualified staff. The preclinical departments in British medical schools, following the trend in the United States, are therefore coming to be staffed more and more by science graduates, who have no clinical experience. The process is already virtually complete in departments of biochemistry (Davidson, 1971), and is rapidly nearing completion in some departments of physiology (Kelman, 1971). Anatomy departments still contain a substantial proportion of medically qualified graduates, but the proportion is falling. Moreover, their supply of medically qualified demonstrators is drying up. The reason is that postgraduate examinations no longer necessitate the acquisition of a thorough knowledge of anatomy, and candidates now prefer to spend their period of study in a pathology department, so attracting an increased salary.

In 1971 the British Medical Association approved the motion 'that because of the serious position with regard to recruitment of medical graduates by preclinical departments, all medical graduates employed in university preclinical and clinical departments should be on the same salary scale'. In the same year the Committee of Vice-Chancellors, which till then, despite repeated approaches, had failed to take cognizance of the situation, decided to elicit some information from the departments concerned. It may be, therefore, that remedial steps may eventually be taken, though they are likely to be too late to avoid a staffing crisis in the near future.

If medically qualified teachers are required, the obvious solution to the problem is to pay them more. The usual argument against this is that such an increase would be unfair to teachers in other faculties. But it can also be argued that the preclinical teacher (whether medically qualified or not) is at a financial disadvantage relative to other science teachers, since he has fewer opportunities of earning money by doing consultative or other forms of outside work. In the year 1968–69 the average university teacher supplemented his salary in this way by nearly 10 per cent, but there was a wide professional scatter about the mean. Thus, professors of social sciences earned an average of £1195 extra, those in applied science £983, and those in pure science £653. The corresponding figure for medical professors was £441 (Bibby, 1970). It is also relevant that both medically qualified and non-medically qualified preclinical teachers often have a heavier teaching load than other science teachers.

SCIENCE VERSUS MEDICINE

The staffing situation in the preclinical departments has consequences of great importance for the future of medical education. 'Pure' scientists, who are nowadays in the majority in the preclinical departments, are not always capable of satisfactory collaboration with the clinicians in combined teaching, nor do they share the common concerns of medical education (Walshe, 1956; Davidson, 1971). The biologist appointed to a department of anatomy on the basis of his experience with the electron microscope may make a poor showing when asked to discuss the anatomy of the inguinal canal with students whose future interest in the topic will relate mainly to the diagnosis of inguinal hernia. Unless he is a particularly broad-minded man, such a teacher may find it difficult to modify his teaching to suit the needs of a doctor rather than those of a scientific specialist (Healey, 1969).

It is not a satisfactory answer to the shortage of medically qualified preclinical staff to call on the services of clinical staff as part-time teachers, though this is sometimes advocated (Christie, 1969). The quality of the teaching so provided is often very poor, since clinical responsibilities often result in lack of preparation or in the last-minute cancellation familiar to all who have adopted this system. Clinical staff may have some value as part-time demonstrators, but only as a bonus, not as a basic asset.

It seems inevitable, therefore, that the preclinical departments must become intellectually and spiritually cut off from the clinical part of the medical course unless something can be done to reverse the trend (Anderson and Roberts, 1965). Already there is evidence of this separation in a lack of understanding between clinicians and preclinicians, and often in a confusion in the student's mind when he is suddenly shifted from one environment to the other. In short, vertical integration [see p. 82] of the curriculum is becoming more and more difficult, and there is a considerable danger of discontinuity between the two parts of what most people still think ought to be a unified experience.

A lack of understanding and sympathy between the two groups of teachers may lead to other kinds of problems. Teachers usually tend to blame the present difficulties of their students on their previous educational experience (as indeed I did in the foregoing chapter), and the clinical reaction to preclinical courses is sometimes distressingly contemptuous. It is still not unheard of for students to be told that they can forget all that nonsense they have been learning and settle down to some real education in the wards. Yet if a preclinical teacher appeals to a clinical colleague for help in the selection of the content of his course he is often told that the clinician concerned feels himself inadequate to interfere. This does not prevent the same clinician from complaining bitterly to other people about the selection which is eventually made.

In most human activities a monetary value is placed upon ability and skill, and some clinicians may thus come to feel that they are superior to those who have elected a preclinical career. It is certainly difficult for someone in receipt of an award specifically labelled 'distinction' not to feel himself more distinguished than his less fortunate colleagues. Yet this 'distinction' does not necessarily apply to his teaching activities, and many clinicians are just as bad teachers and use their time to less advantage than preclinicians.

A further complicating factor is that some clinicians still believe that their duty is to produce a graduate moulded in their own image. There is of course a great deal of truth in this, since the majority of doctors deal with patients in some capacity or other, but it leads to the confident assumption that the clinician knows best what is good for his charges, and this is not necessarily true. From this belief derive the constant complaints received by preclinicians that too little of this or that is taught to satisfy the needs of that or this specialist department, while altogether too much is taught which has no application whatever to the complainant's particular speciality.

PART-TIME CLINICAL TEACHERS

In the clinical years much teaching is done, not by the whole-time university staff, but by the part-time National Health Service teachers. These teachers, who are wholly necessary under any conceivable system for the foreseeable future, are at present doing what is in most cases an admirable job, but they have their own difficulties and problems. Their primary duty is to the sick, and only secondarily are they involved in teaching students. It is thus not surprising that they often have little time for keeping themselves abreast of the general policy of the faculty, and may occasionally find themselves out of step with their whole-time colleagues. The National Health Service consultant who also has a private practice may find it very difficult to programme his time so as to guarantee the continuity of his teaching, and the very nature of his job means that he is not always able to arrange for a substitute to take his tutorials or ward work. The classical example is, of course, the consultant surgeon summoned to an emergency operation 10 minutes before he is due to lecture or give a clinic.

Although some National Health Service consultants and junior staff enjoy teaching and are good at it, others feel it a burden imposed upon them, and evade as much of it as they can. Hence the uneven standards of clinical teaching from one ward to the next and from one hospital to another. Under one regime the student may find himself welcome in the wards and be given a great deal of experience and some responsibility; under another in the same hospital he may obtain only grudging admission to study patients, and as little co-operation as possible.

Departments of general practice are now springing up in the university medical schools and students are being 'farmed out' to general practitioners for training. Many of these general practitioners, faced with the problems of communicating their skills and techniques in an 'apprentice' situation, are finding person-to-person teaching more difficult than they expected, and already courses in teaching methods have been organized for them in various places (Harris, 1970).

TRAINING OF TEACHERS

From what has already been said it is clear that medical teachers, like medical students, are a mixed bunch. Some—unfortunately rare—are born to teach, others laboriously acquire some skill in teaching, and others still have teaching thrust upon them. All have this in common, that at the time of their appointment as teachers they have received no training. School teachers are compulsorily indoctrinated in the methods currently thought most suitable for the instruction of the young, but university teachers never receive any formal course of this kind. They tend therefore to perpetuate the methods and habits of those who taught them when they themselves were students, and this may be the cause of much bad teaching even today. However, many university departments of education now run voluntary courses for junior teachers (e.g. Nisbet, 1967) and it is now being suggested that such courses could be made compulsory. Meanwhile, it is both interesting and encouraging that medical teachers are well to the fore in attendance at them (MacKeith, 1969).

Not much is usually done within the department itself to train newcomers in teaching techniques (Lauwerys, 1950); the head of the department usually feels awkward about advising on such an individual matter, and it may well be that he himself is an indifferent teacher. The matter is thus usually left to the university department of education. In February 1969 a working party on the training of teachers set up by the Association of University Teachers recommended that universities should promote 'regular and purposeful attention within departments to the problems of teaching'. The report suggested that regular reports should be called for from each department, that a senate committee on teaching techniques should be appointed, and that consideration should be given to the appointment of an adviser on the in-service training of teachers.

The voluntary classes run by university departments of education are a means by which new educational ideas, often blown across the Atlantic on the West wind, are conveyed to the lower echelons of the departments in the medical faculty. In consequence there is a certain restlessness and dissatisfaction with current methods of teaching. Until quite recently this restlessness had a minimal effect on the conduct of the curriculum, but in the last 10 years there has been a continual pressure to adopt new ideas, new techniques, new instruments, and new philosophies of teaching. This is the direct result of the increased importance attached to the opinions of junior members of staff. Formerly, the head of a department was himself almost wholly responsible for the methods and content of the courses given in his department, but nowadays, with the growth of other responsibilities, much of the teaching has to be left to the more junior members of the staff, and they are experimenting along new lines. To quote Richard de Bury again: 'In sooth, we who should be treated as masters in the sciences, and bear rule over the mechanics who should be subject to us, are instead handed over to the government of subordinates, as though some supremely noble monarch should be trodden under foot by rustic heels.'

DUTIES OF TEACHERS

These other responsibilities of the senior staff are a very serious handicap to the proper discharge of their primary duties. Before the turn of the century, professors, in common with the clergy, led a peaceful and happy existence. In Scotland at least there was no nonsense about ministers running the women's guild; there were no youth clubs, and no committees to look after the church flowers and the distribution of the harvest festival produce. A good powerful intellectual sermon once a week on hell fire was all that was required.

In exactly the same way, professors of that era were not expected to do anything more than to write one or two books that only one or two people could read, and to get up a series of appropriately incomprehensible lectures; after this their time was essentially their own. Running a department was an easy task, for not much equipment was needed, there were virtually no technicians, and so few students that the clerical work was negligible. In education, as in the church, the situation began to change about the time of the 1914 war, and professors, like ministers, are now expected to do half a dozen different jobs for which they may be wholly unsuited. To an innocent senior lecturer, who at his interview for the chair was asked about only his research work and his hobbies, this comes as quite a traumatic discovery.

The enormous growth of administration in British universities since 1945 is due in part to the increase in student numbers, and in part to the encroachment of bureaucracy on university affairs, for various national and supranational bodies have developed a great interest in how the universities spend their money. Chief among the signs of this preoccupation is a flood of questionnaires. Every few days a professor is expected to answer a detailed list of questions about his departmental research work for the benefit of a different subcommittee of the World Health Organization or for some dictionary of science, and between these efforts he has to make returns to the British Medical Association or to the Vice-Chancellors' Committee specifying exactly how much work of several different kinds has been done by each member of the departmental staff during a selected period. Time and motion study, the final ignominy of the industrial age, has already penetrated university departments, although as yet only in relation to the technical staff.

It is difficult not to unite with Sir Malcolm Knox (1965) in mingled contempt for these time-wasting activities, which appear to be completely useless (Brook, 1968) except as a means of creating work for administrators, and apprehension at the steady encroachment of computerized costing into academic affairs. Many senior teachers, have, in exasperation, given up replying to questionnaires (Russell 1968a), and others may, reprehensibly but understandably, write down the first figure which comes into their heads; a good opportunity for such tactics is afforded by the impossible exercise, demanded by officialdom, of separating the departmental expenditure into research costs and teaching costs. Such a request could only have been made by people with no experience whatever of teaching or research.

But worst of all is the never-ending flow of agenda and minutes spewed out by the duplicators and xerox machines of the army of administrators, both within and outside the university. Professors are now expected to spend something like half their time sitting on committees. The more inoffensive the professor, the more ghastly the committees he is put on (Marshall, 1963). He is expected, no longer to advance his own branch of learning, but to become a half-baked expert on ventilation, student lavatories, computers, closed-circuit television, and the like. He has to decide on assessors for Ph.D. theses written on topics about which he knows nothing. He must on Wednesday give his undivided attention to the revised curriculum for the degree course in biblical study, and on Thursday he must switch his mind to the question of matriculation policy in the eighties.

A few senior academics take to this routine with alacrity, and actually come to enjoy lengthy and inconclusive debates on trivialities and minutiae, rather as Winston Smith came to love Big Brother. Dr. Cyril Bibby has recently and unkindly suggested that they find that such a life 'though wearisome, is less intellectually demanding than either teaching or research'.

Other senior staff react, sometimes violently, in the other direction, and develop their own brand of escapism. Some of the extroverts embark on a series of world tours. If they are not reading a paper in Brasilia, they are attending an International Congress in Tokyo; if they are not on an exchange visit to Bangkok, they are with a committee designing on the spot a curriculum for a new medical school in Basutoland. The papers they give to learned societies in Hawaii do not, as Walshe (1959) has remarked, differ materially from the papers they gave 6 weeks before to learned societies in Prague or Ankara, but their existence is markedly less humdrum than that of the stay-at-homes who are carrying their teaching duties for them. In America, where part-time professors exist, there is a rather bitter joke that the difference between part-time professors and whole-time professors is that part-time professors are actually in their departments part of the time.[2]

The sabbatical year, universal in Australia and in some other places within the Commonwealth, has not yet attained general acceptance in Britain. But even this, sometimes urged as a cure for absenteeism during the 6 years between sabbaticals (Russell, 1968b), is not wholly successful. Surgeons, for example, who are perhaps the most peripatetic people in the medical faculty, stoutly maintain that they must pay visits (usually overseas) to observe new techniques the very moment these techniques are perfected.

Other extroverts become television personalities, and others again adopt the role of outside committee men, and are always in London advising some administrative body or other. Conversely, some of the introverts may take up editing, and spend their time closeted with a never-ending shower of paperwork. A few strong characters simply refuse on principle to attend any meetings whatever.

For these and other reasons, which usually include supervising research projects, writing testimonials, sitting on selection committees, planning the new accommodation which the more gullible expect will at any moment be allotted to them, and innumerable other diversions of a similar nature, the time which senior staff can spend in teaching is limited. In the case of heads of departments it is virtually non-existent—especially for jobs requiring prolonged concentration, such as preparing new and vital forms of stimulating educational experience for the undergraduate students. It seems notably wasteful to choose somebody to be head of a department chiefly on account of his ability as a research worker—perhaps with a sidelong glance at his opinions on medical education—and then to insist on his spending two-thirds or more of his time working as an inefficient committee man. Those who are not so encumbered with administrative duties are in a much better position to appreciate and influence the course of medical education and medical research than those who have

[2] A correspondent to the *Lancet* (1970, **i**, 34), casting round for a suitable collective noun for occupants of university chairs, settled for an 'absence' of professors.

charge of the day-to-day housekeeping of a department and are also expected to take part in running the university's affairs. But such is the perversity of human nature that many junior teaching staff seem to have a compelling urge to throw away most of their advantage by plunging into the millstream of committee work. It is not only students who thirst for power.

John Tyzack and partners, a firm of industrial consultants, who carried out a survey of the administrative structure of the University of Warwick in 1970, reported: 'We have been told that democracy has a special place in university life and that there is constant political pressure from the rank and file of the academic staff claiming the right, not only to be consulted more, but to "have a hand in decision making". The result in practice is already an amorphous and time-wasting system which has led to needlessly protracted argument, dilatoriness in the taking of decisions, uncertainty regarding the effective centres of power and action, and at times to conflicts of policy.' The situation in most medical faculties is not quite so bad as this, since most clinical teachers have sufficient outlet for their altruism and reforming zeal in their everyday work. Nevertheless, the size and inefficiency of medical faculties throughout the country are ominously increasing, and already the laws established by Parkinson in regard to the expansion of work and the coefficient of inefficiency (Parkinson, 1965) are in full operation.

ORGANIZATION OF DEPARTMENTAL TEACHING

Not every staff member has the same skills to the same degree. Some are good at lecturing, some at tutorials: others make excellent demonstrators but are poor at counselling. Clearly the best use of the diverse talents of the teaching staff would result if everybody could be given the job best suited to his particular personality. But this may be difficult because of the pressure of outside responsibilities, and only too often the junior students are entrusted to the care of the junior staff, whether or not they are the people best suited to the elementary type of exposition needed.

A man who has entered upon an academic career in a given discipline should be given an adequate experience in his own department, so that he becomes more versatile, and will in future be able to supervise a department of his own. This means that he should be rotated round the various kinds of teaching being done in the department at intervals, and must be able to obtain help from his seniors in case of difficulty.

Many departments run the risk of becoming inbred. A good student, who performs well in the subject concerned, is invited, after completing his statutory preregistration year, to return to the department on a research grant to work for a higher degree. After obtaining this he is offered a probationary lectureship, and may eventually be promoted to senior status lacking two things—first of all, any detailed knowledge of any medical school other than his own, and secondly, any experience of working at another subject in the outside world.

Such teachers are prone merely to perpetuate the existing pattern of teaching, which is all that they themselves have experienced, and it is very desirable that staff should be drawn from as wide a field of experience as possible. But now that teachers are so difficult to find, this may not be practicable, and in this case it is very valuable if the locally qualified teacher can spend some time observing the teaching and administration of his subject in other medical schools (Sinclair, 1955), for this experience may often spark off new ideas and new enthusiasms.

It is from his seniors that the new teacher should derive the idea that teaching, far from being a dull and unrewarding chore, to be practised in between spells of fascinating and valuable research, is a vitally important activity in its own right. He must learn to be readily accessible to students with problems, even though this means some interference with his own programme, and he must learn constantly to be reading round the subject he is teaching, even though it may appear completely elementary. Failure to do this results in absurdities like those practised in Edinburgh by the third of the Monro dynasty of anatomists, who used to read out his grandfather's lectures word for word, oblivious of the fact that time had moved on in the interval. In short, he must learn that his teaching is just as stimulating and impressive as he himself is willing to make it.

It is also essential that junior teachers in the clinical disciplines should be set a good example by their seniors in their dealings with patients and relations. Students and housemen are among the most imitative of creatures, and the behaviour of the chief has an incalculable effect on their own [see p. 136]. If he is cynical, they become so also; if he is rude, they too degenerate; if he is impatient, his imitators are intolerant and testy. It is not only information which teachers must impart, but a model of conduct; only too often this model leaves something to be desired.

STAFF AND STUDENTS

The ratio of teaching staff to students in British medical schools is still as favourable as any in the world, but some caution is needed in interpreting this ratio, since mere counting of heads can be misleading. In most departments the executive head is effectively prevented from functioning as an efficient teacher by his other duties. Some 'teaching' staff may have research responsibilities so extensive that they play very little part in teaching. Others run service or degree courses for undergraduate science students or supervise Ph.D. candidates.

For such reasons it may be that in a department which appears on paper to have a large staff the teaching of the medical undergraduates is done by only one or two, sometimes fairly junior, teachers. This is particularly the case in the premedical and preclinical years, and especially in departments with a heavy teaching load in the faculty of science, such as biochemistry, genetics, and physiology.

For reasons already given, the presently proposed expansion of student numbers is not likely to be accompanied by a comparable expansion of the numbers of preclinical teachers, and the effective staff-student ratio is likely to fall. It is generally believed that a high ratio allows better teaching because more individual attention is possible, and that students perform better as a result. This contention has never actually been proved. However, it is certain that if the class is small it is possible for the senior staff to get to know each individual and to be aware of his problems. Above a class size of about 60 or 70 this becomes difficult, and though some gifted teachers can carry in their minds the characteristics and worries of the individuals in a class of 100 or so, even they find it impossible with a class of 150, which is reputed to be the minimum economically viable number for a British medical school today.

I cannot believe that the loss of this personal relationship is a good thing. Good teaching is a matter of personal contact of individual minds, and mass production, to me, is its enemy. In a large class, the only staff members who are likely to establish personal relationships with the students are the junior demonstrators, who see them in tutorial groups or in the practical classes. These junior staff, besides being closer in age to the students, also have the advantage that they are free from the suspicion of having much to do with the setting and marking of the examinations. The senior staff, on the other hand, tend to be looked upon as rather frightening father figures, responsible for the failure rate at the end of the year (Ironside, 1963).

Students, like schoolchildren, like to know where they stand, and while it is not easy for a senior teacher in the early part of the curriculum to establish friendly relationships with his students, it is usually possible to command respect. This follows if he takes pains to make his teaching interesting, to make clear how he wants things done, and to insist on a definite standard of performance which is neither impossibly high nor obviously too low. The sergeant-major who drilled me when I entered the RAMC told us, 'There are only two kinds of officers in the British Army, bloody swine and bloody fools'. In university teaching the situation is perhaps not so clear cut, but in the initial stages it is very difficult to arrive at the relationship propounded by the educationists as the ideal—that of senior to junior colleagues. Indeed, this relationship is still an uneasy aspiration in the later stages of the curriculum, though the clinical teachers have an advantage, since by the time they see them, the students are more mature and less suspicious and the atmosphere is less tense, because the misfits have by now mostly been weeded out.

When asked if they have any comments, one of the standard responses students make is that they would like closer relationships with the teaching staff. While this desire may sometimes spring from a lack of self-reliance (Brook, 1968), it is a very reasonable one, which is shared by many teachers. But the big 'impersonal' classes make it difficult to achieve except in small tutorial groups, which will become less and less practicable as the size of classes increases.

STAFF AND STAFF

Finally, a word must be said about the importance of personality. Medical teachers, like their students, are human beings, and as such subject to personal antipathies and friendships. Senior teachers, having been selected largely on their research abilities, are by definition individualists, and may be awkward to boot. These factors, which are often forgotten by those who plan new departures in the curriculum, may render an otherwise excellent scheme of medical education totally useless. If the planners stipulate that every day the students should attend a combined seminar given by the professor of medicine and the professor of surgery, and if the professor of medicine cannot tolerate the sight of the professor of surgery, then the plan will be a failure, however excellent the theory behind it. If the plan calls for a series of physiological lectures to be given in the time allotted to the department of obstetrics and gynaecology, and if the head of this department considers the physiologist concerned to be a charlatan, then these lectures will somehow not be given after the first year or so. These are, of course, perhaps absurd examples, but the best-laid schemes of curriculum committees do often go sadly agley if they neglect a study of the human factors among the staff concerned. It is for this reason that a curriculum which may have been admirably satisfactory when first introduced may fail to satisfy the new teachers, with different ideas and ideals, who are appointed after its inception.

THE DEAN

Until quite recently the office of dean was in most British medical schools a part-time one, filled by one of the senior faculty members for a limited period on an elective basis. But since 1945 the expansion of the medical schools and the development of new educational methods, coupled with the beginnings of control of postgraduate education, have made the task of an unsupported part-time dean virtually impossible. The solution to this problem is not easy, and different schools have tackled it in different ways. Some have opted for the American system in which a permanent appointment of a full-time administrative dean is made; such deans may be appointed to a chair in medical education or some similar post to give them academic status. In other places a permanent whole-time executive dean is appointed to assist whoever is elected to the part-time office of dean, just as senior civil servants are responsible to the minister in the British system of government.

Even with such assistance, the department from which the dean is drawn is effectively deprived of much of his teaching capacity, for so numerous are his administrative duties that he cannot spend more than a fraction of his time in his department (Sinclair, 1955). Many of these duties are not directly concerned with undergraduate medical education, but with representing the medical faculty in the hospital and in the university, as well as with maintaining communications and planning expansion (*British Journal of Medical Education*, 1969). It may therefore be necessary, again as in America, to appoint separate part-time deans to deal with undergraduate and post-graduate problems.

To appoint a permanent full-time dean is to take a major step towards determining the whole future of the medical school, for such a man has considerable powers. If the appointment is successful, all is well, but success cannot be guaranteed, and most full-time deans are very carefully looked at before the post is filled. The system of having an assistant executive dean is less of a gamble in that more controls can be built into the organization; it also has the advantage that the rotation of the deanship every few years allows people from several different departments to gain experience of the running of the faculty.

Vice-Chancellors have been described as persons 'immersed in the practical details of administration, the long drawn involutions of diplomacy, and the delicious bickerings of personal intrigue' (Knox, 1965). This, writ somewhat smaller, appears a reasonable description of the work of a dean of a medical faculty, and clearly a special kind of mind is necessary to excel in it.

4 Medical Schools

In Oxford they ask you what you
think; in London they ask you what
you know, and in Edinburgh they
ask you what the Professor said.
                    Old Oxford saying

BUILDINGS AND PLANT

The third major factor influencing medical education is the environment in which it is undertaken. Many recently established overseas
medical schools possess 'physical plant' which was planned from the
start as a coherent entity sited and composed with the needs of
medical education in mind (Harrell, 1968); the medical centre at
Kuala Lumpur (Danaraj, 1966) is a good example. In Britain no new
medical school was opened between the years 1893 and 1970, when
teaching began at Nottingham, and medical students are for the most
part taught in buildings which have sprung up almost on an *ad hoc*
basis, as money and opportunity became available. These buildings
are usually sited in a cramped and awkward position in the middle of
a large town, where there is no opportunity for expansion, and where
traffic problems undreamed of in the Victorian era make peace and
quiet impossible to obtain. Not only this, but they are often unsuitable
in themselves and unsuitably arranged in relation to each other.

The new medical schools at Nottingham and Southampton should
be more fortunate, for it is proposed to build a medical school/
teaching hospital complex in both places, while Birmingham already
has a medical centre in operation.

Unsuitable accommodation has a greater effect on medical education than may at first be appreciated. For example, it is difficult to
institute a tutorial system in a department which has no space for
tutorial rooms. Again, if the teaching hospital is several miles from
the preclinical departments, a syllabus calling for the students to
divide their time between the two may require careful timetabling,

and perhaps the provision of special transport, if chaos is to be avoided.

The accommodation provided for students is often extremely bad, and so is that provided for teachers (Miller, 1966). Many years ago, when I was occasionally consulted by medical students regarding a possible choice of London teaching hospitals, I used to point out to them that some had many rats and others had only a few. Similar criteria also applied to preclinical departments—for example, there were anatomy departments with elephants, and departments relatively free from them. Apart from these infestations with live and dead fauna, other physical disabilities were, and still are, almost universal.

The first is the appalling inadequacy of lecture theatre design in many hospitals and universities. Some of these theatres are a disgrace to the architects who designed them, and to the heads of departments who allowed the designs to pass. It is perfectly possible to produce a lecture theatre in which the occupants can sit in comfort, hear satisfactorily, and take notes properly, but it is very seldom done. The principles of the anatomical design of seating arrangements have been known for many years, yet they are almost never put into operation. Janet Travell, who conducted a campaign in Cornell University some years ago, produced a number of very effective photographs showing a skeleton attempting to accommodate itself to the totally insufficient distance between the bench in front and the bench behind, and these photographs had eventually some influence on the authorities responsible. Such photographs could be taken in almost any medical school in Britain which has not had its lecture theatres gutted in the last few years. It is difficult to stimulate and inspire an uncomfortable audience, and unreasonable to expect it to take part happily and willingly in new forms of teaching.

In the past it was traditional for each department to have its own lecture theatre, a wholly wasteful situation. Attempts to save space by careful programming of lectures in one central lecture theatre have often foundered because they neglected to provide a first-class air-conditioning system and superlative ventilation. Nothing is worse than a series of lectures sat through in stagnant air and accompanied by a progressive rise of temperature as the day goes on. It is also difficult to convert redundant lecture theatres into other forms of accommodation, and so the existing arrangements tend to be perpetuated.

Small group teaching is a relatively new development in the medical faculty, at least in the preclinical phase, and in the past tutorial rooms were provided on a very niggardly scale; it has proved difficult to insert into already congested surroundings enough of these rooms to meet the demand for this type of teaching. The accommodation for practical class work is often unsatisfactory and overcrowded, simply because of the increase in student numbers in the last 20 years.

This increase has also led to trouble in the clinical curriculum. The old traditional ward round, in which a section of the class followed the clinician round the open ward as he taught on his patients, is now being superseded by the system of bringing the patient to the students rather than the students to the patient [see p. 136]. This system presupposes a suitable room in which such teaching can be done (*Report of the Royal Commission*, 1968), and this is often very difficult to find.

The expansion of student numbers also means that in the clinical years the class is necessarily fragmented; because of the need to exploit as much clinical material as possible, some students have to be sent to outlying hospitals. As a result it is very difficult to assemble the entire group together in one place for systematic lectures. The pattern of teaching must therefore be different from that which is possible when the hospital is large, central, and intimately related to the medical school.

The equipment of most modern universities and hospitals is relatively satisfactory for the traditional forms of teaching, but is often inadequate for newer methods. Overhead projectors are nowadays provided in most lecture theatres, and the standardization of lantern-slides has meant that the many different types of projectors which were formerly necessary can now be discarded. Electrical control of lights and curtains is now almost universal, and most lecture theatres have a public address system. A few have closed-circuit television. But the development of such methods as self-service teaching by means of machines has led to a demand for more and more sophisticated apparatus which in most places is well ahead of the supply. Such methods as the use of multiple tape-recorders linked to automatic slide-changers in pathology museums [see p. 113] are still confined to relatively few schools.

TRADITIONS AND INDIVIDUALITY

It is not only the physical surroundings and the equipment provided by the medical school which influence the teaching within its walls;

each school is more than its component parts, and has its own traditions and its own ethos.

By far the largest centre of medical education in Britain is the amorphous leviathan in London. Not only has London a much greater numerical intake than any other medical school in Britain, it has also had a very different history, and is not a single school but a conglomeration of different units, each with its own background and prejudices. Elsewhere the locus of medical education is the university; in London it is the teaching hospitals. These are not independent 'medical schools' in the same sense as those of the United States, but the network of unity which surrounds them, in the shape of the regulations of the University of London, is fairly elastic, and in some respects the hospitals tend to behave as if they were autonomous. The fiercely individual and competitive traditions which the teaching hospital system has engendered over the years mean that a very great variety of educational experience is obtainable within the university of London. This variety is increased by the extent of clinical specialization, which is not without its pitfalls. It happens, for example, that a student may find himself attached to a clinician whose ward is full of nothing but (say) patients with thyroid disease. When he does his surgical work, he may be attached to a ward full of (say) hiatus herniae. And so on; his progress through the hospital is a progress through successive specialisms. I remember in London in 1938 talking to a medical student who was sitting his final examinations and to my astonishment discovering that he had never been told by anyone that there were four generally accepted areas in which one listened to the heart sounds. This was the direct result of his having been shunted from specialist to specialist without ever having done any general medicine. The problem presented by specialism is greatly diluted nowadays by the use of the large peripheral hospitals associated with London, in which a much greater variety of clinical conditions is available for the student to observe.[1]

But another problem which still exists is the divorcement of the teaching hospitals from the other faculties of the university. Isolation of the medical students is thus inevitable, and it is quite possible for them to go through the entire medical course without ever having established close contact with any other kind of university student.

---

[1] Nevertheless specialism still has its dangers for the student. The rare, atypical, or 'interesting' condition, which tends to gravitate towards the specialist, has a curious fascination for most students, who accord it a wholly disproportionate amount of time and attention (Roberts, 1948).

In Oxford and Cambridge this disability is minimal. Both institutions are organized in a system of colleges, which, like the London hospitals, are highly individualistic, but in which the medical students are thrown together with those in other faculties under common conditions of life and work. But while this advantage—and it is a great one—holds throughout the first stages of the curriculum, in the latter part of it many of the students leave their university surroundings to undertake their clinical studies in London, where isolation from their colleagues is once more a problem. But in any medical school isolation in the clinical years is to a certain extent inevitable; most other degree courses take less time, and the medical student becomes immersed in the professional side of his work while those with whom he entered the university and among whom he may have made most of his friends leave the place to begin their careers.

The medical curricula of Oxford and Cambridge have, in this century, stressed the scientific side of medicine, and in Oxford it is compulsory for the student to take an honours degree in an appropriate subject—usually physiology—before proceeding to his clinical work (Sinclair, 1957d). This science-based degree is, with typical perversity, a B.A. In Cambridge, the Tripos takes the place of this arrangement, but the general atmosphere is similar, and derives from the fact that originally neither of these universities had a clinical school; the medical students had thus to satisfy regulations appropriate to other faculties before leaving them, with a degree, to complete their medical work elsewhere.

Both Oxford and Cambridge operate a fully individualized tutorial system in all faculties, including medicine (Sinclair, 1957d; Badenoch, 1967). This has the advantage that each student is dealt with according to his individual aspirations and abilities, for the curriculum and the educational process can be moulded by the tutor to suit his particular needs. This college-directed arrangement takes precedence over the orthodox curriculum recommended by the teachers in the university departments concerned, who were formerly not always consulted about the sequence in which the student should attend various courses or about the timing of his examinations.

The peripheral schools of England and Wales—those which the London teachers delight in calling 'provincial'—constitute a group which exhibits a considerable diversity, and they differ from those in Scotland in several ways. First, the majority of students in the English schools have had a secondary education on the English pattern, and have gained admission to the medical school by means of passes at the Advanced Level of the General Certificate of Education. In general this means that they have acquired some ability in handling the problems of learning on their own, and also that, in the last couple of years at school, they have directed their minds along circumscribed and well-defined scientific pathways. In Scotland, on the other hand, the tradition has always been to maintain a wider basis for education up until the time of leaving school, and students gain admission to the Scottish medical schools by means of the Scottish Certificate of Education, many of them having little experience of working on their own.

Secondly, the English medical schools admit suitably qualified students directly to the second year of their curriculum, it being assumed that the physics and chemistry and other subjects taken at school satisfactorily covered the ground needed for them to proceed directly to anatomy, physiology, and organic chemistry. In the Scottish schools, until quite recently, it was necessary for entrants qualified by means of a Scottish certificate to take these subjects in a first-year course at the university, no matter how well they might have handled them in their previous examinations.

The situation is further complicated by the fact that the Scottish medical schools have always turned out more medical graduates per 1000 population than the English ones, and an export trade in doctors has been well established for a couple of centuries. The relatively greater capacity of the Scottish schools is now being utilized by many English students, who, if they have suitable 'advanced levels', may be admitted directly into the second year of the Scottish curriculum. The experiment has recently been tried of extending this concession to exceptionally well-qualified Scottish students, but it is perhaps too early to assess the results. At all events the result which is important here is that preclinical classes in Scotland consist of students with different educational backgrounds, and this sometimes causes problems in teaching and in comprehension. Most English schools operate a first-year curriculum for the benefit of those students who for one reason or another have not been able to take the requisite subjects at school, but these departments have nothing like the numbers their corresponding departments have in Scotland. At the time of writing, the universities have been unofficially given to understand that in the near future the Government will no longer provide finance for any such premedical courses, and that the necessary preparation for entry must be undertaken outside the medical school.

At present many Scottish secondary schools are unable to provide the preparation which will be required under this dispensation, and this immediately introduces problems, such as the level of entrance requirements and the possible need to provide remedial and optional first-year classes, which are essentially peculiar to the Scottish medical faculties. Nevertheless, Glasgow has now adopted a curriculum which dispenses with the premedical year of instruction [see p. 68].

Just as the physical plant of British medical schools differs considerably from one university or hospital to another, so their endowments vary. In some places a benefactor may have endowed a chair in a certain subject: elsewhere no such department may exist. In some departments a particularly active school of research may have sprung up and the department may consequently have grown and flourished; corresponding departments in other medical schools may have languished. The teaching capacity of different schools in an individual subject is therefore very variable.

The peripheral medical schools differ considerably in their antiquity. Some, like Southampton, have only just been founded; others, like Aberdeen, have been teaching medicine for a long time. The degree of resistance to innovations may vary correspondingly in different places, and so does the ease with which a new curriculum can be introduced [see p. 164].

SIZE

An interesting summary of the effects of the size of a medical school on medical education within it is given by Hubbard and Howard (1967). In a small medical school, with few students, the class tends to be fairly homogeneous, and can receive much more individual attention from their teachers. There is commonly a strong corporate spirit. On the other hand, staff numbers are small, and the students can therefore be exposed to only a limited selection of viewpoints; the usual shortage of money means that expensive methods of teaching are not practicable and that expensive apparatus cannot be provided.

The large medical school has advantages on the material side and in the heterogeneity of its staff—arguments and discussions are easier to mount where there are many participants to draw upon, and a wider range of technical and professional expertise can be called to the aid of the student. But personal relationships between students and staff are endangered by large numbers, and there is a risk of the more diverse student body becoming disaffected and 'bloody-minded' since they are necessarily treated as statistics rather than as individuals, and are often 'processed' rather than educated [see p. 53].

The current expansion of many medical schools to meet the demand for more doctors is bound, therefore, to alter the character of these schools. It is not possible to share the load of expansion equally among existing medical schools, since, as Walker (1965) pointed out, only those whose cities are large enough can expand without detriment to the needs of clinical teaching. The problem of supplying those selected to expand with sufficient staff, equipment, and money to render the transformation as painless as possible is a very considerable one.

PART TWO

Proposals for Reform

5 Scope and Content of Curriculum

Change and decay in all around I see.
H. F. Lyte

During the medical curriculum the student is expected to acquire information which will help him to understand his present studies and form a basis for his professional work. He is also required to develop skills which will aid his lifelong programme of study and enable him to cope with practical problems in diagnosis and treatment. Finally, he has to develop attitudes which allow him to approach his work with sympathy, tact, and understanding. In this chapter we are concerned with the material content, as opposed to the intangibles, of the curriculum.

QUANTITY

In 1966 George Miller estimated that one new article appeared in the medical journals every 26 seconds, and that the half-life of contemporary medical knowledge was 5 years. Accepting the first of these figures as giving the order of magnitude of the problem, it is quite clear that a lot could be taught to medical students; and it often is. Accepting the second figure (with some caution), it is also clear that much of what is taught subsequently proves to be of little value, and may even be misleading.

Many students, and some teaching staff, complain bitterly about the mental hardship produced by having to learn everything which the curriculum provides, and it is perhaps soothing to remember that students of medicine have always had to know a great deal. For example, as Miller has pointed out, prescription writing in the middle ages was a great deal more complicated than it is today, and there must have been many worries—as indeed there were until just before the last war—about such problems as whether toad's eyes potentiated the action of spider's webs in the treatment of the bloody flux, or whether the two were incompatible. The situation today is not perhaps quite so bad as some would have us believe. Nevertheless, it is undesirable that medical students should have to spend a great part of their working lives in unproductive acquisition of knowledge before they begin to serve the State and earn their own living, and a balance has to be struck between the time for which the State can afford to support medical students (nowadays the medical course is an extremely expensive matter) and the time necessary to fit the student satisfactorily for his future activities in the medical profession. Most students would say of the curriculum, as Dr Johnson said of *Paradise Lost*, 'No man ever wished it longer'.

At present the General Medical Council (*Recommendations*, 1967) considers that the minimum period spent in basic medical education should be 5 academic years followed by 1 preregistration year, in which the graduate works in hospital under supervision [see p. 138]. This view the Council has maintained in spite of some representations that 4 academic years might be sufficient, perhaps followed by 2 pre-registration years instead of 1. At the same time the Council expressed its sympathy with those schools which desired to lighten the examination load of final-year students and to increase the amount of clinical responsibility given to them.

In Scotland the year of premedical studies is still usually taken at the university, making 6 academic years followed by the preregistration year: Aberdeen has moved in the direction indicated by the Council, and has 5 academic years in which the student is formally examined on his work, and a sixth in which he is given greater responsibility and freed from all but clinical performance tests. This system might be described as '5 years plus 2' instead of '6 years plus 1'. A similar proposal is being discussed in Western Australia (Lennon, 1971). More recently Glasgow has introduced a 5-year curriculum in which some of the content of the premedical year [see p. 62] has been omitted, and some has been absorbed into the preclinical teaching.

There is no general definition of what is meant by an academic year. In the medical faculties of most British universities the academic year is longer, and often substantially so, than it is in other faculties. A common pattern is that in the premedical phase the year coincides with that of the science students; in the preclinical phase it is perhaps a few weeks longer, and in the later stages of the clinical phase there may be no more than a month or 6 weeks of vacation time each year.

Nor is the academic week a standard entity. The $5\frac{1}{2}$ day week, each day 7–8 hours long, of formal teaching which could be encountered in some medical schools not so very long ago has been gradually whittled away, and in most places the 'week' is now some $4\frac{1}{2}$ days, each accommodating perhaps 6 confrontation hours. Even this is sometimes an overestimate, for in many curricula there is an unseemly departmental jostling to avoid such hours as 9–10 a.m. (because all parties to the occasion have not properly wakened up) and 2–3 p.m. (because the cerebral blood flow of the class has been diverted to its alimentary canal during the lunch interval). As a result, these unwanted hours sometimes peter out into desuetude and become labelled 'time for directed study'.

For these and other reasons there is considerable variation in the amount of study required of individual students in different medical schools during the 6 years of basic medical education. In the early stages of the curriculum the number of hours allotted to a particular subject bears some relation to the actual hours of staff-student contact, but in the later stages, which depend so much upon opportunity and personal initiative, the hours provided for clinical work have but little meaning.

The Royal Commission on Medical Education (1968), like the General Medical Council, felt that the total time spent in basic medical education could not be reduced, but it did suggest some fairly radical alterations in the ways in which this time was spent. For example, instead of the traditional 2 years of preclinical studies followed by 3 clinical years, it recommended that there should be a 3-year course in human biology, culminating in the award of a science degree, followed by a 2-year course in the elements of the clinical aspects of medicine. This suggestion was made on the basis that 'the essential object of the undergraduate course is to educate the student to university degree standard both in the medical sciences and in the application of these sciences to human diseases'. To accomplish this task the Commission decided that a lengthening of the time devoted to the preclinical and paraclinical aspects of undergraduate medical education was inevitable.

Although the Commission recognized the possibility of considerable individual give and take between the preclinical and clinical parts of the curriculum, some students choosing to include a good deal of clinical material in the preclinical years and vice versa, it felt that the relative emphasis allotted to the two portions of undergraduate medical education should be maintained. Now if a student receives a total of only 2 years of clinical instruction, he cannot be considered fit for independent clinical practice, and this, of course, is not the objective. Even after a year of preregistration study, he will still require a programme of postgraduate vocational training to educate him for his chosen branch of medicine. The Commission's proposals are therefore linked inextricably with an extensive scheme of such training, without which they could not expect to be viable. But this scheme necessarily involves a great deal of organization, expense, and additional staffing, and at present it appears not to be economically feasible. The proposal is thus, at least temporarily, in cold storage.

FACTS AND PRINCIPLES

Perhaps the best of the currently popular educational slogans, one which was nailed to the mast by the General Medical Council in 1957, is 'Instruct less and educate more'. It is based on the need to curtail the immense amount of factual information presented to the student during the years of his basic medical education (Pickering, 1956). The parent slogan has given birth to a family of infant slogans: 'Strip subjects down to essentials'; 'Cut out detail'; 'Teach general principles'; 'Allow students to think for themselves'. All these are, in the abstract, completely desirable ends, and it is only the methods of implementing them which prove recalcitrant.

One of the standard approaches made in the tiresome speeches which infest secondary school prize-givings is to stress that the word 'education' means, not a 'putting-in' of information, but a 'drawing-out' of the inherent abilities and capacity for thought of the student who is being educated. This is at best a half-truth. In the professional faculties of the universities teaching and education are inextricably mixed up, for there is a necessary minimal basis of fact which must be included in the curriculum, though nobody can define its limits. The 'essentials' of a subject are not always the same as its 'principles', and factual information must be imparted throughout. The distinction between a general principle and a detail, though it sounds impressive, is often extremely difficult to make, and the safest general rule is that general principles are taught in your own department, and details are taught by other people.[1] Very few teachers can recognize a general principle when they see one, and no student can deduce a general principle

[1] Pickering (1968) concludes that fundamental principles are similar to basic prejudices, except that the first are approved and the second disapproved: each represents a hypothesis with which you approach a new set of data.

unless he is provided with a satisfactory factual basis to work from.[2] In fact, in the study of the human body, principles or laws are few and far between (Roberts, 1948). As a student, I was taken by the phrase, 'Attend to the emunctories', which occurred several times in my textbook of medicine. This indeed appeared to be one of the few general principles I have personally encountered, but what did it mean? In the dictionary I found that emunctories were excretory organs, but how in practice ought I to 'attend' to them? A little detailed instruction would have stood me in better stead than a single woolly principle.

It is impossible to delete technical details from the curriculum, for the ideas on which medicine is based cannot be taught without giving illustrative examples, and essential information cannot be understood except in a setting of supportive factual material. The philosopher Chuang-tzu, a disciple of Lao-tzu, maintained that nothing is useless. As he pointed out, a traveller who is crossing a plain *uses* only the portions of the plain which are directly beneath his feet. Yet if the rest of the plain were suddenly abolished, either his unsupported footholds would crumble away, or else he would lose his nerve and fall off into the abyss.

Facts, then, are inescapable, but we could certainly reduce their numbers, provided we could recognize which ones can be dispensed with and which must be retained. It is here that the slogans fail us utterly. What *are* the 'essentials' of any given subject? There is no agreement on this, even within the department concerned in teaching it, and it may be instructive to consider the experience of Greulich (1953). In response to criticisms of the length and content of the anatomy course, Greulich asked each of the critics to enumerate the things they wanted properly taught to medical students by his department. It transpired that, if all the requests were acted upon, the course in anatomy, far from being shortened, would have had to be extended for a full additional year.

For many years now anatomy has been the universal target for shafts of wit and abuse concerning the teaching of detail (Martin, 1957; Sinclair, 1957c, 1966). Much of this criticism has been singularly ill-informed, for it stemmed from the personal experiences undergone by the critics when they themselves were students. As Meadow (1970) said, 'Our image of any branch of medicine other than our own is the vivid image which excited and alarmed us when

---

[2] Dr. Arnold of Rugby was said to be so addicted to enunciating principles that, if he was confronted with a case that could not be immediately classified, he would at once invent a new principle to cover it.

we met it for the first time as students, many years ago. We all forget that while our own field has changed for the good in the last 10 years, so too have others.' To many senior doctors the emotive words 'anatomical detail' or 'topographical minutiae' conjure up a vision of the course and relations of the greater petrosal nerve, or the vascular anastomosis in the middle ear. But such things have not been taught for years. The General Medical Council (1967) must be suspected of falling into this trap when it says that 'detailed topographical anatomy is best regarded as a subject for specialist vocational training'. What is 'detailed topographical anatomy'? Is the conducting system of the heart,for example, a specialist matter? Or the relations of the appendix? Or the lymphatic drainage of the breast?

Now that anatomy courses have been so much curtailed [see p. 75], it is likely that the other preclinical subjects will come in for abuse. On the wall of every preclinical student's room is to be found a chart of the Krebs cycle and its ramifications; in the drawer of his desk is another showing the interrelationships of the structural formulae of the steroids. Above the shaving mirror is the hexose monophosphate pathway, and inside the back door, above the coat-hook, is the mathematical derivation of the theory of the sodium pump. When taxed with teaching 'biochemical minutiae' or 'biophysical detail' the biochemists or biophysicists tend to reply that nobody knows what may be valuable in 10 years' time. This is perfectly true, but, as the anatomists have been repeatedly told, it is no excuse for teaching it now. The General Medical Council is at pains to recommend that education should continue throughout the life of any doctor, and if some omitted biochemical topic does become vital in 10 years, then surely it can be given in refresher courses for those who need it.

Similar considerations apply to each of the other departments contributing to the content of the curriculum, but the choice of material to be taught ultimately devolves on the teaching staff of that department, who are likely to err on the side of liberality with facts and principles. The usual device the faculty adopts for limiting the amount of detail taught by the battery of experts with whom it has to deal is to cut down the teaching time of each department. This is done purely on the basis of the sum of the prejudices of the members of a committee brought together for the purpose. Each department is usually asked what amount of time it would consider reasonable; this figure is then divided by the number the committee first thought of, and the department concerned is left to make the decisions on what to teach and what to leave out in the time available [see p. 74].

This procedure, admirable for departments strong in prestige or influence, tends to operate to the detriment of the smaller and weaker departments according to the law reported by St. Matthew (Matt. 13:12).

George Miller (1962) investigated the range of time available for each individual subject in American medical schools. If all the maxima had been incorporated in the same curriculum, the students would have had to work, assuming a 40-hours week and a 40-week year, for a total of 4 years and 7 months to complete the requirements. If another curriculum had included all the minima, the students would, under the same conditions, have had to work only 1 week over 2 years. Miller stresses that the time spent in the curriculum is not the essential factor; the crux of the matter is the performance of the student at the end of it. 'In the end it matters only what a student has learned, not what he has been taught.'

DEAD WOOD AND NEW BROOMS

Another powerful educational slogan is 'Cut out the dead wood'.[3] This is relatively easy in the clinical part of the curriculum, for new and more satisfactory methods of treatment and diagnosis automatically displace older and more unsatisfactory ones (Arnott, 1949). The recognition of the cause of a disease in itself deletes a great quantity of speculation. Preventive medicine constantly eliminates diseases which were formerly taught in detail.

In the preclinical part of the curriculum, however, it is not so simple to cut out dead wood. This is partly because it is more difficult to recognize it; it is almost impossible to predict which aspects of a subject like biochemistry, which is growing exponentially, will be relevant to the practice of medicine in 10 years' time, and which will be useless. In the circumstances, the reaction of the department is, very sensibly, to try to retain as much as possible of what it considers to be 'fundamental' knowledge. However, a great deal of this knowledge will prove totally valueless to the practitioner of medicine. Similarly, in anatomy it is impossible to say that a detailed knowledge of any given part of the body will not prove useful at some time or another in the course of medical practice. It is thus very difficult to select a 'basic' course from the material available, and, as we have

[3] An earlier version was given by Sir Thomas Browne: 'To purchase a clear and warrantable body of Truth we must forget and part with much wee know'.

FBE

seen, no two clinicians agree as to what is professionally essential and what is not.

At curriculum committee meetings it is often argued that what the student should receive is a careful grounding in the scientific aspects of each discipline he encounters. It is agreed that the objective is to produce a scientifically based graduate, and it is claimed that such a graduate cannot 'understand' the material he is taught unless he is taught it in the same way and in the same depth as a science student. It is true that medical students have such a broad education that they tend to get a very superficial view of the various disciplines they sample, and there is no time to allow them to dig deeply to obtain a proper understanding of any one of them. In contrast, the science students have a narrower range of studies, and may spend several years in the pursuit of knowledge within a single discipline.

The proposal that medical students should undergo a similar sort of education is often heard, particularly in departments where the staff contains no representative of the medical profession [see p. 43]. It is natural to think that those studying your own subject are best educated by the sort of methods to which you yourself were subjected. Yet I believe this attitude to be wrong. It is quite possible to plan a very satisfactory course while keeping always in mind the ultimate objective of medicine rather than science, for there is very little difference for purely educative purposes between professionally useful and scientifically useful material. However, it is difficult for people who have no medical degree to recognize and select professionally valuable material.

Many preclinical and premedical departments therefore take the view that it is up to the clinicians to tell them what they want taught. Here, then, is another source of disagreement and argument [see p. 71] at faculty meetings. Until new methods of assessment have been developed to tell us whether students educated in one way are better able to perform satisfactorily in certain directions than students educated in another, it seems that the problem is insoluble.

Critics of the orthodox British curriculum have for some years maintained that the contributions made to it by different disciplines were out of balance when considered in relation to the requirements of current clinical practice. Not only this, but the course was too inflexible; every student had to go through the same programme, whether or not he was going to use the material afterwards. Thus, the future physician learned too much anatomy, the future orthopaedic surgeon too little; the embryonic pharmacologist required much biochemistry, and the intending radiologist virtually none. Again, all students were required to spend the same length of time in clinical clerking, though the gifted student might get as much information and experience in a much shorter time. If he attained a satisfactory standard earlier than his more average colleagues why should he not be allowed to spend the time so saved in following his own bent in another clinical direction? (Roberts, 1948). The feeling thus began to gain ground that there must be, embedded somewhere in the excesses of the orthodox curriculum, a central core of material suitable for all types of students, who could then build on this foundation as their particular needs dictated. This point of view is complicated by the constant pressure from 'new' subjects thought to require time in the curriculum, for any such encroachment, if the total time spent in medical education is not to be increased, is necessarily at the expense of time allowed to the existing subjects.

The prestige of a department has always depended on the amount of teaching which it undertakes during the course [see p. 12]. But an additional new reason why each department should do as much teaching as it can manage to secure is that nowadays the best way to make a case for obtaining additional staff is to teach large numbers of students for as long as possible. The extra staff thus merited can then undertake research, which in turn attracts funds and so contributes towards the growth of the department and its capacity to claim additional teaching time. This spiral staircase towards fame and fortune is an excellent reason why empire builders should squabble over the allocation of teaching time. Meetings of curriculum committees thus frequently become acrimonious, with the 'haves' aligned against the 'have nots', and have indeed been said to resemble battles between feudal states.[4]

The outcome of these battles depends, regrettably, upon the algebraic sum of the prejudices of those concerned in them, and on the amount of support which can be whipped up beforehand. At present the structural sciences are under general attack, and the educational pendulum has swung away from anatomy and morphological pathology towards biochemistry, biophysics, psychology, and sociology. More and more time is being ceded to the chemically based aspects of medicine and to the social sciences, and anatomy, in particular, has been in full retreat for some years past.

The decrease in anatomy teaching time is indeed the most spectacular of the recent changes in the content of the curriculum, and has

[4] 'It would seem to me,' said Pickering in 1956, 'that the main problem of medical education is this: will the medical course be arranged primarily in the interests of educating the student, or primarily in the interests of the prestige of the teachers?'

not only cut down the amount of factual material taught, but altered substantially the type of training the student's mind receives [see p. 28]; the effects of this are—like the effects of most curricular changes—unknown.[5] In 1953 the mean number of hours allotted to anatomy in British curricula was 960 (Sinclair, 1955), but by 1965 it was 580, 6 schools having 500 hours or less. In 1970 the figure had fallen still further, and a proposal (now superseded) was made that in the Glasgow curriculum anatomy should be restricted to 276 hours.[6] In America the process of anatomy-baiting has proceeded so far that there is already a call for remedial courses for those who have been unable to cope with their clinical work because they received inadequate grounding in the subject (Skandakis and Gray, 1969; Healey, 1969); in Britain the diminution of emphasis on the morphological aspects of the human body means that those who intend to specialize in such careers as surgery, orthopaedics, or radiology will need postgraduate courses in anatomy to fit them for the practice of these specialities. It may also be that postgraduate refresher courses in anatomy will be requested by general practitioners, who are liable to find that their knowledge of anatomy is inadequate to deal with the day-to-day problems they meet in their consulting rooms (Hines, 1970). At present no obligation is laid on any university department to provide such teaching.

Anatomy, which in the last 15 or 20 years has served as a quarry of teaching hours from which inexhaustible amounts of building material for other empires could be extracted, has now reached a stage beyond which it cannot be worked at a profit, and other existing disciplines must, therefore, come under attack from the newcomers, and, indeed, from their older-established colleagues. Who, then, are the newcomers, and what of the material which is being incorporated into the curriculum?

Most of the new disciplines which already have a foothold in the curriculum and are attempting to extend their boundaries within it are scientifically rather than clinically based. Examples of these 'new' subjects are genetics, statistics, biophysics, sociology, and psychology, and their expansion produces a tendency for the curriculum to become slanted more and more towards the science, and less and less towards the art, of medicine.

[5] Ironside (1963) stresses the psychological impact of opening up and dissecting the body, and concludes that the medical student must have plenty of time to learn anatomy so that he can make the necessary adjustments within himself. If the time is too short, the adjustment 'will be the defensive one of active forgetting'.

[6] Miller (1971) considers that 'ambulance man's anatomy is an appropriate basis on which to begin clinical instruction'.

The General Medical Council (1967) suggested that 'instruction should be given in those aspects of the behavioural sciences which are relevant to the study of man as an organism adapting to his social and psychological, no less than to his physical, environment. Instruction in the biological and sociological bases of human behaviour, normal emotional and intellectual growth, and the principles of learning theory should be included'. The Royal Commission on Medical Education (1968) was of the opinion that 'far too little attention has generally been paid hitherto to the study of the behavioural sciences'. There is thus nowadays considerable pressure to include a substantial amount of social science teaching in the curriculum, and it is pertinent to inquire how this has been, and is to be, done.

University departments of sociology and psychology are at the moment under considerable pressure because of the immense growth of student interest in these subjects—a growth which is part of the drift away from the physical sciences, but which is also encouraged by the widespread student impression that they provide 'easy options' for indifferent students, who do not have to work so hard as they do in the physical or biological sciences or in the traditional arts subjects. The staff, are, accordingly, not well placed to take on still further teaching responsibilities, or to spare the considerable amount of time needed to formulate the best possible service course for medical students. Existing courses for medical students given by departments of psychology are often presented, sometimes very badly, by junior members of the teaching staff, and the material they contain is ill-chosen for the needs of the medical student. Psychology has been so busy establishing itself as a science that it has acquired a preoccupation with rats which tends to stamp itself on all elementary courses in the subject. Such material, though fascinating in itself, is not the best preparation for clinical work, and medical students often acquire an ill-founded contempt for the subject as a whole (Davis, 1970). If the additional hours to be allotted to psychology are to be similar to the ones already in operation in many medical schools, then nothing but a time-occupying lesion will result. Yet it would be perfectly possible, if senior psychologists had the time and the interest, to establish a very meaningful, important, and practical course for medical students (Platt, 1965, 1967).

A common solution to these difficulties is to entrust the department of psychiatry with the responsibility of giving instruction in elementary psychology, and this usually results in a more relevant selection of topics. But the fact must be faced that the interests of most psychiatrists lie more in the direction of clinical psychiatry than of basic psychology, and the course which they mount may not be wholly satisfactory. Indeed, in many curricula psychiatry is itself a rather untried newcomer, and it was only in 1967 that the General Medical Council gave it the status of a major clinical subject, pervading the instruction in all types of illness; not all medical schools in Britain as yet support a chair of psychiatry (*Report of the Royal Commission*, 1968).

The problem of providing a satisfactory course in psychology thus remains for future solution (Pritchard, 1970; Davis, 1970), and the Royal Commission's report sums the matter up: 'By and large, current teaching in the behavioural sciences to medical students is sketchy, either too lightly or too heavily influenced by clinical interests and poorly related—if at all—either to the other preclinical sciences or to normal human behaviour as experienced by the student.'

Sociology is much more of an unknown quantity than psychology, and one which many members of medical faculties view with undisguised concern. Just what is the student going to get out of a course in sociology that he would not acquire in any case in his passage through the orthodox medical curriculum, which often contains a course in social medicine largely slanted in the direction of sociology? Maybe he will obtain something of great value, but this has not yet been demonstrated, for the content of such courses has not been subjected to detailed evaluation and criticism.[7] The Royal Commission makes many general suggestions and comments about instruction in the behavioural sciences, but until these have been acted upon for some years there will be no means of assessing just how they work out in practice. Another problem is that many sociology departments appear to set their sights at a low academic level, at least in the junior classes, and, because of the enormous demand on their services, contain staff with little teaching experience. The standard to be required of the medical students in a course provided by such a department is therefore a matter for some anxiety. Yet the Royal Commission considers that teaching in sociology, as in psychology, should be given 'in close contact with the main stream of scientific interest within the university' rather than by the resources available within the medical faculty. The medical faculty is, in fact, being asked to give what amounts to *carte blanche* to the social sciences in order to see what they can do for medical students.

---

[7] The only course in behavioural science about which fairly full details are available is the pioneer first-year course in psychology and sociology at Edinburgh, which has been in existence since 1964 and occupies 130 hours (Martin, MacPherson, and Mayo, 1967). Hooper (1968) has described another substantial (88-hour) course.

But it is not only new subjects that are anxious to replace anatomy as the doyen of the preclinical sciences; there are contenders for the job among the existing disciplines. Chief among these is physiology. The Physiological Society (Denton and Phillips, 1965) has already put in its claim that physiology is the only subject with 'sufficient content and relevance to medicine' to lay a proper intellectual foundation for the professional maturation of the student, provided that it is studied 'over a sufficient period'. It is clear from the wording that the period at present allowed is considered to be far from 'sufficient', and there are those who would like to see the orthodox preclinical curriculum, often described (with occasional venom) as 'corpse-centred' (Denton and Phillips, 1965), exchanged for one which might with equal justice be termed 'cat-centred'.[8]

Another educational lobby at present in the ascendant is that which bases itself on molecular biology. Although Burnet (1971) has recently challenged the value of molecular biology to medicine, either now or in the immediate future, this is an unpopular view (Harris, 1971), and the seemingly inescapable trend is for more and more information of this kind to be imparted to the medical student. Indeed, molecular biology has been pressing its claims so hard and so vociferously that many people are now in danger of forgetting that such a thing as a whole organism exists (Denton and Phillips, 1965). Nobody can deny that ultimately the whole of medicine will prove to be founded not merely on molecules but also on subatomic particles. However, an excess of such basic material, which even its protagonists have to admit has little *immediate* application to clinical medicine, inevitably displaces other, more pragmatically useful, data. Much more important is the problem of deciding how much biophysics, biochemistry, genetics, and cellular biology should be taught to medical students in the elementary stages of their career.

It is perhaps here that the greatest difficulties arise in the selection of material to be taught. It is the contention, for example, of many pharmacologists that students must have enough biochemistry to understand in detail the actions of the drugs which they prescribe, and if this were completely accepted it would necessitate a very considerable course in biochemistry. But a great deal of structural biochemistry as at present taught is quite irrelevant to this objective, and indeed incomprehensible to practising consultant physicians.

[8] 'I have heard highly-intelligent scientists say: first, that electronics ought to be one of the most important subjects in the curriculum; second, that a knowledge of the anatomy of the cat is far more useful and important than a knowledge of the anatomy of the human. These remarks were not made lightly but with complete seriousness by otherwise highly-intelligent and sensible men' (Pickering, 1968).

Secondly, new drugs are introduced and put into use at a rate which virtually precludes the non-specialist from keeping up with the biochemical theory behind them. Not all the actions of such a familiar substance as insulin are understood, and its structure was not accurately known until quite recently. Is it seriously suggested that nobody should use a drug until he completely understands its chemistry?

Just the same, the enormous advances made by pharmacology and therapeutics in the years since the war obviously necessitate a considerable expansion in the amount of undergraduate instruction in these subjects and in their chemical basis. The growth of microbiology and chemical pathology also requires underpinning by biochemistry, and the permeation of preclinical and hospital work by biophysical methods and concepts has made a case for extending the instruction in this subject.

Many other alterations in the distribution of time among the various subjects in the curriculum are currently taking place, and it would not be profitable to pursue them in detail. Psychiatry is expanding, and so is instruction in community medicine[9] and general practice; statistics is being encouraged by both the General Medical Council and the Royal Commission. Such changes in emphasis are inevitable, and often seem desirable, but nobody knows, or makes any attempt to find out, their effects [see p. 160]. In a matter which affects so many careers, and possibly even so many lives, it is surely essential to examine every change very carefully. This is particularly so in cases where changes seem to be proposed for the sake of change itself, in response to pressure from untried sources, or as a result of the subjective intuitions of those with an axe to grind, whether they be students or teachers.[10]

INTEGRATION AND CO-ORDINATION

Integration

Some critics of the orthodox curricula, both in Britain and in America, felt that a system which exposed the student to a succession of 'subjects' studied in different departments was wasteful (because

[9] Nobody knows what community medicine is, but the Royal Commission feels it to be a 'Good Thing' (Jefferys, 1969; Logan, 1969).
[10] As Samuel Butler put it, 'The wish to spread those opinions that we hold conducive to our own welfare is so deeply rooted in the English character that few of us can escape its influence.'

of unnecessary repetition), disjointed (because of isolation from other 'subjects'), and confusing (because of departmental differences of opinion). They pointed out that the student who dissected the stomach in his anatomy course might wait some months before he learned about the control of its secretion, a year or more before he entered the pathology department to discuss the matter of peptic ulceration, and perhaps 2 or 3 years before he saw a gastrectomy and was taught about the clinical results of vagotomy. This was claimed to lead to a disunity in the student's mind, since he was never presented with a complete picture of the stomach in relation to medicine, but only with a series of overlapping snapshots, taken from different angles, and separated from each other in time.

Further, many believed that those students who were attracted to medicine from a sense of idealism found themselves discouraged and stifled by the premedical–preclinical–clinical sequence of instruction. It was, they claimed, difficult to maintain a sense of vocation and of duty towards humanity while studying the wilder tracts of genetics, statistics, or biochemistry without having been given any idea of the possible applications of the information being taken in.[11]

These feelings first found expression in the distinctive contribution made by the educational experiment at Western Reserve University (Patterson, 1956; Caughey, 1956) in the early fifties, and from one aspect of this experiment derives the magic word 'integration' which has dominated medical education for 20 years. In this time a very large number of man-hours has been devoted, in different places, to the devising of integrated curricula. It is important to be clear about what is meant by 'integration', since some medical schools, climbing upon a swiftly moving band-waggon, have failed to read the destination indicator on the front.

The word 'integration' is applied to a system in which departmental barriers are completely broken down, and the content of the curriculum is presented by staff acting under the control of 'topic committees'. The committees, not the departments, devise the programme, to which teachers from the individual departments concerned contribute as directed. The essential feature is the subordination of departmental interests to a committee on which the department is usually, though not always, represented.

The original programme put into action at Western Reserve was based on what is now called 'systematic' integration. The student,

[11] It is also educationally wasteful to neglect the strong motivation towards learning provided by the romantic fantasies with which many medical students approach their subject matter (Miller *et al.*, 1961; Strassman, Taylor, and Scoles, 1969).

instead of progressing from one department to the next, or from the study of the normal to that of the abnormal, studies in sequence the systems of the body as they are presented by committees whose members are drawn from the preclinical, clinical, and often the premedical departments. Every aspect of each system is treated in its entirety before the next system is considered. The student may dissect a lung one morning, study the pathology of emphysema that afternoon, and next morning see a postmortem on a case of lung cancer, followed by a discussion on the sociological aspects of cigarette smoking. When the respiratory programme is finished, he proceeds to another programme, perhaps on the genito-urinary system, which is treated in the same way. The rationale of this method of teaching is that it overcomes the separation in the student's mind between the form and function of the system concerned, its diseases (including their social and preventive aspects) and their diagnosis and therapy.

'Horizontal' integration means that two or more departments teaching concurrently merge their educational identities in a course controlled by a committee. Thus, in the preclinical part of the curriculum an integrated course in human biology [see p. 86] may be substituted for the orthodox courses in anatomy, physiology, and biochemistry. The working parties planning a school of medicine and human biology recommended a clinical course not artificially broken down into 'subjects', and the General Medical Council (1967) suggested that the student should be introduced to medicine and surgery 'less as separate disciplines than as different facets of medicine in the wider sense'. (To implement this idea adequately requires a revolution in the present practice of departments of medicine and surgery.)

In contrast, 'vertical' integration means a similar collaboration between two or more departments which normally teach seriatim rather than together. For instance, there may be an integrated course in the physiology and pharmacology of the alimentary canal; the departments of anatomy and paediatrics may collaborate to give a vertically integrated course on human growth, and those of physiology and medicine may combine to present an account of lung function.

The potential advantages of both methods are obvious. It is only too common to find that a student who can discourse satisfactorily on the arrangement of collagen fibres in connective tissue has completely failed to connect these fibres in his mind with the collagen he has been studying (even in the same week) in the department of biochemistry; the information is recorded in two separate textbooks, or in two different sets of notes, and he never thinks of collating the two. Again, it is often only by seeing the abnormal that the student is led to understand the normal. For example, it is much easier to appreciate what is meant by the distribution of a peripheral nerve after examining the results of a peripheral nerve lesion. Even minor degrees of preclinical-clinical collaboration, short of true integration, can be extremely valuable. When a particular system is being discussed in a preclinical department, a visit from the appropriate clinician may illustrate the importance of the structural and functional material which the student is learning. Unfortunately, not every clinician can adjust himself to the level of instruction required, and some find it difficult to avoid clinical details which may not be understood, or may be seized upon at the expense of the lesson intended.

At the end of an integrated course comes an integrated examination in which the student has to write integrated answers to integrated questions; the material presented in the course is treated as a composite whole and is not in any way subdivided according to the component disciplines involved.

This, in very brief outline, is the concept of integration; it aims at giving the student a holistic, instead of a fragmented, outlook on his studies. Some institutions, however, have, like Humpty Dumpty, determined to make the word mean what they want it to mean. Until quite recently, for example, most premedical curricula contained separate courses in botany and zoology. Some of the material in these courses, particularly the formal descriptive botany, was felt to be unsuitable for medical students, and most schools decided that they should be taught only those aspects of both subjects which served the needs of the medical faculty. Accordingly, a new subject of 'biology' was substituted, and this is often called an 'integrated' course. However, all that commonly happened was that zoology was cut down to two terms and botany to one, with a certain amount of consultation between the two departments. The examinations at the end contained botany questions and zoology questions, with no attempt to examine the work as a composite whole. To call such a course integrated is a complete misuse of the word.

The question of the integrated examination in fact often proves a stumbling block. Teachers who are quite willing to submerge their departmental identities in a general pattern of instruction may find it impossible to relinquish their belief that the student must pass an examination specifically devoted to their own particular 'subject' before he can be certified as fit to proceed with his studies. This at once destroys the whole concept. Where there is an attempt to integrate subject A and subject B, and A insists on a separate 'subject' examination, then the student merely brings with him two notebooks; in one he writes down the information he judges to belong to A and in the other the material he considers to belong to B. When the examination in A draws near he takes out the appropriate notebook and works from that. It is useless to provide an integrated course if the examination pattern makes the student disintegrate the material again into its component 'subjects'. British students, in an examination-orientated society, will certainly do nothing to jeopardize their chances of promotion.

This highlights only one of the many administrative difficulties inherent in an integrated course, of whatever sort. If one of the essential contributors will not 'play', the whole thing collapses. The more people there are whose co-operation is required, the more likely is it that someone will be included whose heart is not in the project, and who will make his own reservations as time goes on, even to the extent of disrupting the work of others.

The second main snag is the considerable additional staff effort and organization which such courses entail. In the orthodox system, once the curriculum and the timetable have been decided, the administration of the departmental teaching becomes an internal matter; lectures and practical classes can follow each other as is most convenient, and can be planned so that they occur regularly, at set times. But the demands of integrated teaching are difficult to reconcile with departmental routine. Thus, the lectures and seminars to which the department contributes may be separated from each other by irregular intervals, so that it becomes difficult for the staff member to remember his responsibilities, and difficult for the department to keep track of him. The result is that unless a skilled and conscientious administrator is specially appointed to implement and supervise the programme, there is a considerable risk that staff members will fail to turn up to vital sessions, that preparations will go wrong, and that chaos will ensue. The more links in the chain of communications, the more likely it is that one will break.

In the Western Reserve experiment the topic committees originally scrutinized every piece of information presented, and this was found to be extremely expensive of staff time. Yet unless it is done, repetition and disagreement will once more arise. If combined methods of presentation are used [see p. 112], and they are essential to such courses, rehearsals are necessary to make sure that all the desired points are properly covered.

Systematic integrated courses are thus difficult to mount and to administer, and initial enthusiasm for them may wear thin fairly rapidly. Indeed, they tend to die out 3 or 4 years after their initiation, as new junior staff are appointed and the enthusiasts leave for other posts. Systematic integration also suffers from the basic defect that it merely replaces one set of discontinuities, confusions, and repetitions by another; for what are the laboriously planned 'system courses' but new 'subjects' in disguise? Under the old dispensation the student used to learn the physiology of all the systems of the body in close sequential proximity, and gained a grasp of how they interacted with each other; he lost, perhaps, some understanding of how pathology modified their functioning or how pharmacological intervention affected them. Under the new dispensation he studies the physiology of one system at a time, along with its anatomy, pathology, and clinical aspects. He gains in seeing how all these fit together, but he loses by not obtaining an idea of how each system interacts with the others.[12] The separation in time between the treatment of the structural, functional, and clinical aspects of a given system in the orthodox curriculum is matched in the integrated curriculum by the separation in time between the programmes dealing with two systems which intimately affect each other—for example, the cardiovascular system and the urinary system. Another problem is presented by the growing intellectual and professional separation between the teachers in the preclinical and clinical phases of the curriculum [see p. 44]. In the old days there was no need for vertical integration, considered as a special teaching device. Vertical integration was the job of every clinician (Marshall, 1956b), for he was considered capable of putting together the fragments of information from each and all of the basic medical sciences as they became necessary for the understanding of the clinical conditions under consideration. Nowadays the growth of specialism has rendered the clinician, through no fault of his own, incapable of sustaining this function without help, and the rapid expansion of the preclinical sciences is bound eventually to make vertically integrated teaching sessions a more and more demanding intellectual exercise for both types of teachers concerned.

The General Medical Council (1967) recommends that 'the relevance to clinical problems of Anatomy, Physiology, Biochemistry, Psychology, Sociology, Pathology, Microbiology, and Pharmacology

---

[12] Normand Hoerr, who was professor of anatomy at Western Reserve during the period of upheaval, maintained that the greatest loss under the new system was the ability to visualize and comprehend the body as a whole.

should be illustrated throughout the whole period of medical studies'. This will become progressively more difficult, and the best solution probably lies in 'topic teaching' sessions to which preclinical scientists are invited (Roberts, 1967); at least this kind of vertical collaboration would maintain some contact between the two parts of the curriculum.

The concept of integration has given rise to two opposing views of the curriculum. The first, which stresses horizontal integration in the preclinical stage, is that medical students should begin by taking a science degree course in 'human biology' (a course in 'regulatory mechanisms', as it is called in one prospectus). This composite discipline replaces the traditional courses in anatomy, physiology, and biochemistry, and may also include material drawn from the disciplines of ecology, anthropology, genetics, statistics, biophysics, psychology, and sociology. In 1963 the working parties which reported on the possibility of founding a school of medicine and human biology stipulated the content of such a course in some detail, and the Royal Commission on Medical Education (1968) adopted a similar, though less detailed, syllabus[13]; a third proposal is that of Tanner (1958). Burnet (1964) suggests five divisions of human biology (at the levels of the species, the individual, functional anatomy, cellular dynamics, and molecular biology) which should be taken by every student, with provision for study in depth of any one of them.

The development of such horizontal integration, complete in itself, could provide a very satisfactory course for science students, and could also allow for the introduction of an honours year from which medical scientists could be recruited. But the system inevitably produces a schism between the preclinical and the clinical teaching. The punctuation mark of the science degree reduces the possibility of concurrent vertical integration, and does nothing to lessen the feeling of many students that they are being fobbed off with science while what they want to do is to heal the sick.

In direct conceptual opposition to this scheme is the idea of encouraging as much vertical integration as possible, so that from the outset of the curriculum the student is treated as a potential doctor, rather than as a potential medical scientist. The objective

---

[13] '. . . the origin, evolution and geographical deployment of mankind; the growth of human populations and their structure in space and time; human development and heredity; the properties of the human genetic system and the nature and import of the inborn differences between individuals . . . human ecology and physiology and many of the aspects of human behaviour that are the concern of sociology and cultural anthropology . . . the nature, origin and development of communication between human beings and the non-genetical system of heredity founded upon it.' It is perhaps significant that no mention is made of the structure of the human body in this prescription.

here is to prevent the loss of enthusiasm and idealism which is common if the first part of the curriculum has a purely scientific slant [see p. 81]. There is no reason why a certain amount of horizontal integration should not be combined with this approach, but the resultant difficulties are just as great as if systematic integration is being practised. For this reason, although either of these opposing schemes has its attractions, what is probably not very satisfactory is the sort of compromise between them that some medical schools seem to be attempting.

Co-ordination

However, if the ideal of integration is replaced by the less demanding ideal of co-ordination, matters become a great deal simpler. Under the orthodox system each department is left completely free to organize its teaching in the way that suits it best. The anatomy department might therefore discuss the cardiovascular system and dissect the heart at the same time as the physiology department is giving a course on the central nervous system, and the biochemists are talking about protein metabolism. In a co-ordinated system of teaching, each department is still left to determine the content of its courses and their internal details, but it is asked to co-ordinate the sequence of its teaching with those of the other departments, so that the same topics are dealt with at about the same time. At first sight this appears difficult to organize, since, for example, physiology has a great deal to say about body fluids while anatomy has virtually nothing to contribute on this topic. However, it is possible to arrange a co-ordinated course so that the study of structure always precedes that of function (Sinclair, 1958, 1965b), and so that the discrepancies between what each department is talking about at a given time are reduced to a minimum [see APPENDIX]. The advantage of this method is that each departmental course is complete in itself, and consists of lectures and practical classes given at set times every week. There are thus no administrative difficulties beyond the initial ones encountered during the planning of the course. By such simple means it is possible to make the teaching more coherent and meaningful, and it is also possible to interpolate integrated discussions, debates, and symposia, since each department will have been considering different aspects of the same theme, and can therefore collaborate efficiently in such presentations. The General Medical Council (1967) has expressed itself in favour of such interdisciplinary 'topic teaching'. A co-ordinated course may with considerable profit be followed by an integrated examination [see p. 83], which makes the student combine and correlate the information presented to him, and affords him a most useful exercise.

Curiously enough, difficulties may arise over the co-ordination of teaching within a single department. In the department of anatomy, for example, it was formerly common to find the content of the lecture courses divorced from that of the practical work in the dissecting room. This situation originally arose because unsatisfactory methods of preservation rendered it desirable for the body to be dissected as quickly as possible, some students having to work on the lower limb at the same time as their colleagues were working on the head and neck or abdomen. In most anatomy departments the process has now been rationalized so that everyone dissects the same part at the same time, and the lectures can be tied to the practical work. In other disciplines, however, the separation of lecture material from practical work is still a problem. By their nature, physiology practical classes demand the use of expensive equipment, and as a result it is common to try to save money by rotating the class in small groups through a series of set experiments. In consequence, each group has a different educational sequence of experience, which is not complete until the whole cycle has been gone through. It is therefore difficult to avoid giving lectures which, for many of the groups, are unconnected with their current practical work. Similarly, it is virtually impossible to programme a system of clinical lectures which fits in satisfactorily with the experience obtained by each individual student in the wards.

Whatever methods are adopted, and whether integration or co-ordination is the objective, it is vital for both staff and students to realize that the students must play an active part in the success of the venture. The important thing is that the student has to pull the various aspects of each topic together in his mind. This is the main educational value of such teaching, but many students find the greatest difficulty in doing it; it is for this reason that integrated courses in the early stages are less successful than those in the later years of the curriculum.

THE INTERCALATED YEAR

It is the aim of all university teaching, in whatever faculty, to bring the student to think for himself, and critics of the orthodox medical curriculum have pointed out that the student was swamped in a morass of detailed factual information; so many different disciplines claimed a share of his attention that he had no time to find out what any one of them was really about. The admirable slogans 'Encourage initiative', and 'Give them time to think' are directed against this situation.

As usual, difficulties arise over the translation of these slogans into practice. How is the student to be made to think for himself? How is his initiative to be developed? And how can he obtain the experience of finding out something of the doubts and uncertainties which underlie even the most dogmatic of the statements in his textbook?

One solution, which is a feature of many curricula, is the provision of an intercalated year. The student is allowed to step aside from the direct path of his medical studies to spend a year pursuing some problem or topic in greater detail than is possible in the necessarily superficial general medical course. Usually it is specified that this experience cannot occur unless his performance has been better than average in the classes taken during the first 3 years of the curriculum. The experience, in other words, is not a right, but a privilege accorded to the better students.

In some places the work he does during this extra year consists mostly of extra study within a given discipline or disciplines; in others the year is spent entirely on a small research project carried out under supervision, and in a third group there is a combination of both activities. The experience of more profound study of a given subject must undoubtedly benefit the thoughtful student, who may by this means be brought into a much more critical frame of mind, and encouraged to read round the subject and to question the pronouncements he encounters as he does so. To tackle a small research project of one's own is to gain an insight into the difficulties of obtaining a straightforward unequivocal answer to any biological problem, and a healthy and critical attitude towards new developments in medicine and science. Both methods thus result in an increase of the critical faculty and a willingness to examine data more carefully; this can do nothing but good (General Medical Council, *Recommendations*, 1967). As against this, the student takes an extra year on his shoulders in addition to the already formidable number of years intervening between the time of entry to the medical course and the time of financial independence.

The subjects studied during the intercalated year will naturally vary with the student's inclination and the degree of enthusiasm for this kind of teaching displayed by the individual departments. The

Physiological Society (Denton and Phillips, 1965) makes a good case for studying physiology in some depth, and the other popular subject in most medical schools is pathology. However, any subject can be suitable for the purpose intended provided the student is allowed to come to real grips with it. Ellis (1967) has suggested that there are good reasons why students might find it more profitable and enjoyable to study a clinical subject, and in Monash University it is possible for them to do so (Dudley, 1970).

Intercalated years are rewarded by an intercalated degree—in science, medical science, or medical biology, according to the local terminology. For students at the top of the class, with intelligence and drive, the experience is clearly a good thing, and the degree is probably a help to them if they wish to obtain certain types of employment after they graduate in medicine. Nevertheless, it is interesting that few of them appear to choose a career in the pre-clinical sciences, let alone the particular science in which they chose to work for their intercalated year. It is also interesting that few of those who combine their medical course with an honours degree in one of the preclinical sciences seem to make an academic career in the corresponding preclinical department (for an example see Davidson, 1971).

The recognition of the benefits which this system can offer to the more gifted students has led a few schools to the conclusion that what is good for the few must also be good for the many, and they have made the intercalated year compulsory for everyone. But very few students are capable of getting the best out of an intercalated year, and to hold the less gifted ones back from completing a perfectly satisfactory medical degree, in order to make them flounder around trying to master some small aspect of a particular subject, is both unnecessary and unwise. In Oxford, for example, where the structure of the degree system demands that everybody should read for an honours school, every medical student is compelled to take an intercalated year, usually in physiology. At the end of this he emerges, sometimes a wiser man, but sometimes with that contradiction in terms, a third- or fourth-class honours degree, and just as much confused by his experience as benefited by it (Sinclair, 1957d).[14]

In other places attention has been drawn to the fact that students in the medical faculty spend a great deal longer time in the university than students in most other faculties, and the curious concept has

[14] The new medical school at Southampton proposes that the whole of the fourth year of the normal curriculum shall be spent in 'study in depth' (Acheson, 1969).

arisen that in the clinical years their very seniority should be recognized by a degree.[15] Such a degree, it is additionally argued, allows the student who discovers he is not fitted for clinical work to leave the medical course with something of value to him in seeking other employment, whereas if he receives nothing to mark his achievement in lasting out 3 years or so he is no better off than if he had never started. These ideas involve the award of a medical science or medical biology degree to everyone who satisfactorily completes the first 3 years of the curriculum. Such a degree is thus a hand-out for no additional work, and there may be little enthusiasm among the students for it, even though it was instituted in their interest. When everyone receives a distinction, it ceases to be a distinction, and students may even refuse to graduate with their new letters, holding them not to be worth the paper they are written on. 'When everyone is somebody,' said Gilbert, 'then no one's anybody.' Curiously, very few indeed of the students to whom it has so far been awarded seem to make use of it for the purpose intended—by leaving the medical course and taking up a job for which the degree was of some value.

PROJECTS

Less drastic than the intercalated year, but with the same objective of encouraging initiative and personal interest, is the practice of handing out projects. Such projects, which are now a feature of many different kinds of education, represent attempts to make the student think for himself and to gain experience of working on his own. With the best students they may be—even spectacularly—successful, resulting in publishable work (Liebow, 1956), but many students do not want projects, and regard them as merely another chore which has to be got through with as little trouble as possible. It might be said, without too much distortion, that the bottom two-thirds of the class get very little out of the project system, and that the top one-third do not need it anyway.

Projects impose a good deal of extra work on the staff, and are perhaps the most difficult method of instruction to use effectively (Miller et al., 1961). It is difficult to devise suitable projects for perhaps 150 students, and the inevitable result is that some turn out to

[15] This is actually urged by the Royal Commission on the grounds that medical students would find it 'irksome' not to have a degree when science students doing courses of human biology have the status of graduate students after an essentially similar course.

be too short, while others are gigantic, occupying every waking hour and some months of vacation time. It is usually fatal to allot a project and leave it at that; most students require help, and virtually all will balk at the task of writing it up unless they are continuously stimulated to produce a report. It is therefore often a full-time job to see that all the reports are returned on time. Like essays, projects are often included in intercurrent assessment schemes [see p. 147], and the difficulty of comparing and evaluating a large number of different projects, dissimilar in difficulty and intrinsic nature, is very considerable. Only too often the project is neither returned nor criticized.

In some places combined projects are assigned to groups of students, who must then break down the problem into its components and allot the components to individuals—a method resembling the procedure in practical classes of the same nature [see p. 131]. In others a central project committee allots the projects, while in others still the student merely chooses the department in which he would like to do his project, and decides the details with the head of that department.

However the matter is arranged, it is necessary to allow adequate time for the completion of the project; in some places the project is a spare time activity, and in others a certain number of hours is set aside each week as 'project time'. All this complicates the timetable, particularly when specially 'fancy' projects are being undertaken.

OPTIONS AND ELECTIVES

A further move towards a variable curriculum which can be adjusted to individual needs is provided by the introduction of optional courses. The student is allowed to choose some classes which he himself would *like* to take, as opposed to the classes which he *must* take. For example, some students may wish to take extra physiology in order to extend their knowledge of physiology beyond the elementary level which it is possible to achieve in routine teaching for the whole class. Or they may wish to learn something of histochemistry, which is usually not taught in detail in the routine histology class. This idea is relatively new in Britain, but in America it has been a commonplace for many years in such medical schools as Yale (Sinclair, 1955). It involves every department in arranging one or more 'elective courses' for the students to choose from, and these may be easy or difficult to stage-manage. Usually the time available for them is short, and this may easily result in the production of 'snippety' courses, the value of which is doubtful. The additional problem of formal assessment of such courses also arises, for unless they are examinable some students tend to regard them as an excuse for doing nothing.

Another difficulty is that in the early stages of the curriculum very few students have thought much about their future career. They have a vague idea that they would like to be doctors and heal the sick, or that they want a safe, secure and well-paid job, but they do not know whether they are to be radiologists, physicians, experimentalists, or hospital administrators. It is therefore impossible for them to make a reasoned choice of activity in their first couple of years at a British medical school, and any elective chosen at this time must naturally be selected on the basis of pure prejudice (often derived from some-one else). Mistakes in selection will therefore be common, and it is for this reason that elective courses are usually restricted to the later stages of the curriculum.

It is also true that electives are not equally valuable or easy to arrange in all departments. A busy department of biochemistry, with enormous commitments to the faculty of science, may find it extremely difficult to provide any electives more elaborate than a course of library reading and an occasional demonstration. It is clearly impossible for them to encourage medical students to undertake some kind of research elective, since at this time in their career students require almost total supervision, and the time and apparatus is simply lacking. On the other hand, some physiological or anatomical techniques are easy enough for students to learn and to use to some purpose in quite a brief period.

Despite these difficulties, the Royal Commission has recommended the adoption of a 'flexible course structure' in the first 3 years of its suggested curriculum. This course is based on the award of a degree following the accumulation of a specified number of 'modules', or 'course units' in different subjects or parts of subjects. The Commission suggests a core of compulsory modules, surrounded by a group of 'limited alternatives', which is in turn surrounded by a group of 'options' among which the student has a completely free choice. Such a structure, as the Commission points out, resembles many university courses in the United States and elsewhere, in which the student can take a selection of 'units' and pile them up, one on top of the other, to make a little tower of achievement. Provided this tower is of the requisite height and does not contain too many bricks of unacceptable colours,[16] a little flag representing a degree may be planted on the battlements, and the new tenant is presented with an imposing certificate which he can use as a meal-ticket.

To make matters even more difficult, the Commission suggests the inclusion of remedial modules in the premedical subjects and in mathematics, to allow those students who obtain insufficient grounding in these subjects at school to make up the necessary leeway. They also propose the possible inclusion of clinical modules or formal instruction in clinical matters. Finally, they suggest that many of the modules offered should be available to students other than medical students, and that the course should be followed by a degree, either in science or in medical science, according to local preference.

CULTURE

As an extension of the principle of electives within the medical faculty, some critics are now demanding, in the name of the sacredness of the individual, an opportunity for students to follow their own bent, whether or not this involves material directly relevant to the medical curriculum. This demand stems from the belief that the medical student is less 'cultured' than his colleagues in other faculties. This belief, which has no experimental foundation [see p. 16], has led to the application of the principle of elective choice to courses within other faculties of the university. It seems, in fact, as if the core of stipulated medical achievement recommended by the Royal Commission on Medical Education is on its way to being regarded by some people as less important than the opportunity for the student to do as he wishes.[17]

Because of the suspicion (no more) of comparative narrow-mindedness, it is urged that medical students should have the opportunity of taking courses in Spanish, in mediaeval history, in business management, and so on, as part of the requirements for their medical degrees. While a case could be made out for almost any individual subject of this kind, the taxpayer could also inquire with

[16] In many places the process of acquiring a degree by combining units such as botany, physiology, logic, astronomy, and radiobiology is known as stamp collecting.

[17] At least one self-service curriculum exists in America. Since 1968, students at Yale have been allowed to work out their own highly specialized courses of study in the last 18 months of the curriculum. 'If a man wants to co-ordinate his individual course with medical jurisprudence or with applied engineering, he will now be able to do so.' (*Medical News*, 16 February 1968.)

some cogency just why it was necessary to spend his money in this way. In other professional faculties no such theory is at present advanced, though of course the curriculum for a law degree has always recognized and tolerated a certain amount of general 'culture'. However, engineers, dentists, and theologians must be watching the progress of this idea in the faculty of medicine with considerable interest.

I personally do not believe that medical graduates are any less cultured than their colleagues in other faculties (the arts graduate is notoriously narrow-minded outside his own field), and even if they were, I do not think that this is a proper way to acquire 'culture'. If a student's interests lie in the direction of classical music, he can attend musical courses in the evenings during his medical studies. He can obtain gramophone records from the library, and he can take lessons in his spare time. I do not believe it is justifiable to suggest that he should take music classes as an integral part of the requirements for his medical degree. Nevertheless, the pressure for such concessions seems to be spreading.

However, there are difficulties. In the first place, very few arts or science courses can be suitably fitted into the medical curriculum, and unless virtually the whole class elects for the same subject, special courses can never be provided, for the arts and science faculties are just as hard pressed for staff and time as is the medical faculty. The suggested 'free' choice thus boils down to a very few alternatives which happen to fit in with the timetable. Again, supposing these problems to have been overcome, every student coming up for assessment at the end of the year may have had a different educational experience. How are they to be assessed? Some of the 'outside' options are 'soft', and some may be extremely hard. Many students may have made the wrong choice; they may have thought they were interested in Aramaic or statistical geometry, but when they actually come to study the subject they find that their interest is rapidly extinguished. If this is the case, they may well fail their examination in the elective subject. How is such a student to be disposed of? He has passed satisfactorily all the subjects required of him by his professional mentors, but has failed in his elective because he made an ill-informed or unsuitable choice. Is he to be extruded from the medical course because he failed in Hebrew? Or in computer programming? In some places the administrative difficulties posed by such situations are solved by not requiring the student to take an examination in the outside subject. This appears to me to make the situation worse. Either the course is essential for the student's education or it is not. If it is not, and it is possible to give the required amount of professional material in the medical course in a shorter time, why do we not do it? It would be much less expensive, and those students who wished simply to obtain a straightforward medical education would be able to graduate more quickly.

If a student is desperate to obtain 'culture', there are many sources available to him. He can attend classes at the nearest technical college, he can work in the vacations in the library or at some job which bears on the material he is interested in; he can take a correspondence course; he can attend art galleries and museums in his spare time. Those very few students who genuinely feel that they are being cheated of an adequate cultural environment by embarking on a medical course are surely capable of fending for themselves in their reading, their listening, and their viewing. No nation in the world is so well catered for in respect of culture by their broadcasting service.

The question of culture can be dealt with in other ways. In some places there is an official and compulsory 'cultural subject' embedded in the first-year curriculum. This subject, which may be English, mathematics, logic, or another similar course, is programmed in exactly the same way as the other subjects; the examination must be passed. The student, who tends to regard the course as merely extra examination material, is likely to acquire a distaste for it similar to that which so many children acquire for authors compulsorily studied at school. The basic assumption underlying this sort of arrangement appears to be that culture is something which can be picked up in a briefcase and carried off as a life's companion. With a truly stimulating instructor it is possible that sparks might be struck from tinderboxes in the minds of some of the medical students, but first-year classes of this kind are usually given by junior instructors, and my own small experience of them is such as to suggest that the student would acquire from them very little culture, but a great many indigestible facts and opinions which he would find it necessary to regurgitate at the examination.

Elsewhere there are optional alternatives. For example, a Scottish student who has been exempted for one reason or another (perhaps by an excellent performance in one of the Certificates of Education) from one of the premedical subjects of the medical curriculum, may be permitted to substitute an approved alternative, providing the timetable allows this. The main difficulty here is again the question of assessment.

The fact is that culture cannot be enforced. Like wisdom, it is something intangible which is acquired insensibly during the course of other activities. If we can only succeed in the objective of teaching the student how to use his own mind, culture will become automatic, and each student will reach out in the direction which he finds most interesting and satisfying.

FREE TIME

By free time, properly speaking, is meant time entirely within the control of the individual student, in which he can do exactly as he pleases. It is therefore not to be confused with time left free for electives or projects. For example, a student may be said to be allowed 'free time' to undertake a piece of library research. But this may have been specified by his tutor, and he may be required to deliver a talk upon it to his colleagues. Such time is not properly 'free', and a distinction must be made between the two concepts.

Free time, as an educational technique, was introduced in America to counter the effect of the excessive amount of factual material given to the student in the ordinary medical curriculum every day. As a result of the weight of this material there was no time to study anything outside the set routine, and the provision of free time allowed a needed breathing space in which the students could set their ideas in order, and for the first time view the material they had accumulated with a degree of understanding.

This idea must be seen in the light of the considerable differences between American and British students. In the first place British medical students are seldom so overloaded with material as their American colleagues (Cohen, Hughes, and Richardson, 1957), and the lurid picture which some educators appear to have of student academic requirements—a picture in which from dawn till midnight the student staggers round from lecture to practical, from seminar to clinic, and from library to postmortem room, till at last he falls senseless into bed—is not in accordance with actuality, though it is an article of faith with many of the students themselves. Secondly, the American 'free time' was intended to be used by mature students who had already been through a college degree course before taking up medicine. They were thus in a position to use their free time to the best advantage, to develop, as the proponents of the idea hoped, their own habits of thought, their own ideas, and their own initiative. In a mature adult, with a high intelligence quotient, a high drive to succeed, and a basic urge towards the practice of medicine, this may well be true. But in an immature 18-year-old student in this country, its chances of success are small. Given the afternoon off to think, most British preclinical students gravitate towards the billiards table in the students' union or to the golf course. Instead of reading up the literature of the subject, pursuing and perfecting their clinical technique, or writing original papers, they may take their girl friends to the cinema or their cars to pieces. Many students in British medical schools have had no previous educational experience to fit them for the proper use of free time, and are singularly devoid of the inner fire which alone can make a success of the idea. Even in America not every student uses free time to the best advantage. Colwill (1969) considers that while the 'more outstanding of the students showed a striking tendency to utilize free time for educational purposes . . . for weaker students portions of free time might very appropriately be used for remedial educational activities'.

However, matters improve as the students become older and more responsible, and in the later stages of the curriculum they may make quite good use of judiciously interpolated periods of free time. Even in the early stages it is possible to effect some improvement in the general attitude by providing guidance as to how the time should be used. Demonstrations, conferences, discussions, and debates may be set up, which, although not examinable, serve to attract the students' attention in suitable directions. Later, they may utilize their free time to write up case notes, to study their clinical cases, to visit their patients at home, or to do some library research. Even then, however, it is a great help to most students to have some assistance from staff members regarding the most suitable form of activity.

Most students have an immense ignorance of how to learn and of which methods of learning are likely to suit them best. They may also be quite unaware what they are learning the material *for*. It is often very useful to have 'free-time' seminars at which various careers in medicine are outlined, or in which laymen give their experiences of various occupations which the medical graduate may have to understand when he qualifies. Such sessions may be organized by the student societies, which sometimes welcome the opportunity to hold meetings during free time instead of in the evenings, when attendances are usually lower.

If free time is introduced into the curriculum, it is important to programme it rationally. A 'free' hour from 12–1 p.m. every day is, for example, virtually useless, since it may take half an hour for the student to switch his mind off what he has just been doing, and he can only just get started on his free-time occupation when he has to break off for lunch. It is probably best to allow free time to accumulate so as to provide a free afternoon or morning every week. In the Western Reserve system this concept was extended so that $1\frac{1}{2}$ days a week were left free, and the student could accumulate the free time with a view to spending it away from the medical school (Boake and Epstein, 1958).

STUDENT TRAVEL

It is traditional that travel broadens the mind, and nowadays in the summer vacation the transatlantic planes bulge with their cargo of medical students intent on this objective. Cheap student fares, travel grants and concessions, and faculty encouragement for this sort of thing have all increased the traffic beyond recognition. Student exchanges take place between far distant medical schools, sometimes for a term, sometimes for a year; vacation work in overseas hospitals is recognized for certain faculty requirements, and preregistration posts abroad are allowed.

Much of this activity is excellent for broadening the mind, and some of it is good for medical education also. A glimpse of how medical matters are arranged elsewhere cannot but be stimulating and thought-provoking (Whitehead, 1952). But it does sometimes happen that the trip degenerates into a glorious orgy of travel on a Greyhound bus, a marvellous holiday, a collection of colour transparencies. This is a result not unknown to those who attend overseas postgraduate conferences or symposia, and it is possible that, like such gatherings, subsidized student travel can be overdone.

The British Medical Students' Association has an organized scheme for facilitating student travel by providing information about temporary appointments, both in Britain and overseas: it arranges inter-university exchanges and study tours, and can help to a limited extent with finance. The BMSA is apprehensive that with the curtailment of the summer vacation in the clinical period of most medical curricula the opportunities for travel and exchange may diminish in the future (Ekeid, 1966; Garraway, 1969).

6 Acquisition of Information, Skills, and Attitudes

> If you'll only let the children alone
> and not always be meddling with
> them.
>
> *Lord Melbourne*

ORGANIZATION OF TEACHING

A very great deal depends on the way in which teaching is structured —that is, on the timetables of the various 'subjects' and the alternation of teaching methods. It is clearly undesirable to have one lecture immediately following another, or to have gigantic 4-hour practical classes in the same subject. The Royal Commission Report (1968) recommended that the planning and control of the curriculum should be taken out of the hands of the heads of individual departments and become the duty of an interdepartmental committee. Such a committee inevitably faces considerable resistance from reactionary heads of departments, and undertakes an extremely difficult job when it attempts to formulate a timetable [see p. 170].

In the preclinical part of the curriculum the education of medical students must be fitted in with the education of science students, who have extensive commitments outside the departments concerned, and it may prove impossible to achieve the ideal arrangement suggested by the Royal Commission, that the teaching of each department 'should be concentrated into a single day, or two days, in each week, so that the staff can be freed for research and other work during the remainder of the week'. From the same circumstances derive the occasional horrors of planning, as when it becomes apparently inevitable to have three successive lectures in places separated from each other by a mile or more [see p. 57]. Most of these can be got round, but difficulties remain, and it is a fortunate school that is able, in the preclinical years, to follow the advice of the Royal Commission that there should be 'no more than about two hours of formal teaching in any one teaching day, and at least one hour should be used for seminars: the remainder of each day being taken up by practical work, demonstrations, discussions and reading'.

In the clinical years the claims of patient care and outside committee work make for other problems. Over two-thirds of the students surveyed by ASME (*Report of the Royal Commission*, 1968) felt that they had been bored or inadequately occupied at some stage during their clinical course, and much of this is attributable to periods of standing round, doing nothing, waiting for a clinical teacher to turn up to his scheduled class. The best timetables cannot eliminate this sort of thing, but a system of organized substitutes would help, as would an encouragement of the feeling that clinical teaching is a basic responsibility of those who undertake it.

TEACHING AND LEARNING

In the minds of many educational reformers 'teaching' seems to be equated with an essentially passive transference of information through exposure to such traditional exercises as lectures, films, and demonstrations. It is contrasted, to its detriment, with the active process of 'learning', in which knowledge is acquired through experience of practical and clinical work, discussion and debate (Bligh, 1970). Evidence quoted in support of this supposed dichotomy includes the Chinese proverb which runs: 'I hear, I forget; I see, I remember: I do, I understand', and the usual proposal made by the reformers is to cut down as much as possible the passive methods and multiply the active ones. This is often encapsulated in the slogan, 'Make them use their own minds'.[1]

There is a good deal of truth in the suggestion that, *as practised* by staff and students, certain methods of teaching are more passive than others, but it does not follow from this that they cannot be made to demand a great deal of individual mental effort on the part of the student. Again, *as practised*, many so-called 'active methods' are much less satisfactory than their proponents would like to believe. It is always essential to make a clear distinction between the possibilities of a teaching method and the way in which it is commonly put

[1] Millar (1962) rightly points out that we should be more concerned with the ways in which students can acquire knowledge and how they utilize it than with the details of the content of the curriculum.

into action. Because there are many bad or indifferent lecturers and few good ones, it does not follow that lecturing is necessarily a bad or indifferent way of teaching (Netsky, 1960; Dunlop, 1962). Because there are few good medical films it does not mean that films and filmstrips are therefore of little use. Rather, it ought to mean that the full potentialities of these methods should be explored, so that they can be brought to greater general efficiency, and only then should their place in the curriculum be judged.

In 1964 the Committee on University Teaching Methods, set up by the University Grants Committee under the chairmanship of Sir Edward Hale, published a report in which the opinions of students on various teaching methods were synthesized with those of the teaching staffs to achieve a balanced evaluation. Although the faculty of medicine was not included in this survey, many of the findings in regard to the other faculties are very relevant to the medical curriculum. But the best source of information and advice on teaching methods and materials is probably *Teaching and Learning in Medical School*, which contains contributions from the School of Medicine and the School of Education at the University of Buffalo (Miller *et al.*, 1961). The advantages and disadvantages of various methods of teaching are analysed from the point of view of the objectives desired and the results attainable, and the book could be read with profit by every medical teacher. Another most valuable survey is that of Beard (1970), though this is not specifically concerned with medical teaching.

THE SPOKEN WORD

Lectures

Lecturing as a means of instruction has a history extending back before the introduction of printing. In the past it was widely respected as an important source of information and inspiration, but nowadays attempts are being made to discredit lectures as being out-of-date and of very little value (e.g. Hopson, 1967; McCarthy, 1970). It is perhaps odd that many of those who take this line are often to be seen attending postgraduate lectures, and are themselves not averse to visiting medical schools overseas to give a course of these same old-fashioned sessions. As Dickinson (1953) put it: 'For our students, we have thrown the lecture into outer darkness, as an outworn remnant of an earlier pedagogic era; but for ourselves, we teachers continue to lecture to each other, almost incessantly. We dash all around the country, indeed half way around the world, winter and summer, leaving our appointed tasks—such as teaching students— and when we get there, what do we do? We sit down and listen to lectures, or, worse still, we stand up and give them.'

It is undoubtedly true, as Dr. Johnson pointed out, that lectures were more valuable in the days when textbooks were scarce, badly written and badly illustrated. Nowadays, when the quality of books is so much better, it is a waste of time for the lecturer simply to repeat or paraphrase material which the recommended books contain, but it must be admitted that there are still lecturers, in the faculty of medicine as in other faculties, who do just this. To read from one's notes or from a book, as well as being totally useless, has a disastrous effect on student morale (Cohen, 1950). On the other hand many students, even in the Welfare State, are unable to buy every book that is recommended, and the library often cannot provide enough copies of them to satisfy the demand.

Different subjects lend themselves to different proportions of lectures and other forms of teaching. To take one example, topographical anatomy is best learned in the dissecting room, for the regional arrangements are essentially visual material, and to talk about them in words is less illuminating than to see and feel them in three dimensions. In contrast, much of the course in genetics can be handled by means of lectures.

Lectures may profitably be used in two ways (*Hale Report*, 1964). The first is to provide a basic framework for the student, indicating to him the scope of the subject, the sources from which he can obtain information, and the ways of thought involved in it. In this, the usual system, tutorial classes or seminars are used to fill out the lecture framework, to help the individuals in the groups with their problems, and to allow them to question and discuss along the lines which they themselves find most interesting and profitable.

The second way of teaching is the reverse of this, in which the basic framework teaching is given in tutorials or seminars, and the student is advised to attend such lectures or other classes as his tutor feels are suitable for his individual abilities and interests. This system is much more restricted in its distribution, and finds its fullest expression at Oxford and Cambridge (Sinclair, 1957*d*). In other universities, although a staff member may have several students allocated to him as a 'regent' or an 'adviser' [see p. 139] he seldom has the power to control the detailed programme of any individual student.

To give a course of lectures, as the Hale report points out, is considered to be an honorific or responsible task, and some teaching staff feel it a reflection upon their ability if they are not asked to do so. Accordingly, there is a considerable danger that too many lectures may be given, and this is undoubtedly common in the medical curriculum.

The drawbacks of lectures as a mode of instruction have often been listed. Inevitably, they proceed at a level too simple for a few students and too difficult for others—some therefore become bored and others confused. Personal contact with the students is minimal, and no satisfactory discussion is usually possible; the teacher receives little 'feedback' from the class. If a student is ill, he misses what has been said for ever, unless he can borrow a garbled version of it in the shape of his neighbour's notes. Students are very critical of the quality of lectures; they ask for fewer and better lectures, closer staff-student relations, and more teaching in discussion groups (*Hale Report*, 1964).

On the other hand, lectures have advantages. One of the greatest of these is that the whole class can be exposed to the same material at the same time. The set books do not always run exactly parallel to the ideas of their recommenders, and a lecture course may be very successful in imparting the shades of emphasis which are locally considered desirable. A lecture can cover more ground than a seminar, and do so in a more logical and better thought-out fashion, for preparation is possible with a lecture, whereas a seminar must be spontaneous if it is to be useful [see p. 110]. A lecture can also be more timely than the textbook, which is of necessity out of date (Sinclair, 1956b), for the lecturer can bring the students right up to the advancing edges of the subject in hand. He can indicate impending developments; he can put his own individual interpretation on matters of doubt or difficulty; he can explain, at greater length than is possible in the set book, material which the student may not understand; he can exhort, stimulate, impress, and enthuse his audience. Unfortunately not everyone can do these things, and dreary and pedestrian lectures are all too common (Meredith, 1950). Yet this does not invalidate the technique, and a skilled lecturer can be most valuable (Sinclair, 1955; Williams, 1969).

A course of lectures can never hope to cover a subject completely, and this is a very difficult thing for inexperienced and immature students to understand. This is perhaps especially so in Scotland, where there is often a greater dependence on intellectual spoon-feeding in the early stages of the curriculum than there is elsewhere.

The Scottish tradition (Dunlop, 1962) has until now been in favour of completeness and exactness in lecture courses, and some students still attempt to take down every word which the lecturer says in the belief that this, and this alone, is the material which will get them through the examinations. In England students are rather more relaxed, and a few actually attend lectures without taking any notes at all.

Quite apart from the routine lectures forming part of the curriculum, students are often invited to lectures given by peripatetic scientists or clinicians. When a visitor comes to a medical school the first reaction of his hosts is usually to ask him to give a lecture for the benefit of staff and students. The incurable desire of distinguished medical graduates for expense-free travel leads to an almost inexhaustible supply of such lectures, and on every medical faculty notice-board are to be found intimations of departmental, faculty, and even university lectures of this kind. These are always *added* to the existing lecture programme, and never substituted for it. Particularly in the clinical years, the circuits within the students' minds may thus be overloaded by continuous high-voltage instruction.

Lectures of this kind may be good, fair, or catastrophic. Not every visitor is an expert lecturer, and the difficulty of pitching his talk at the right level is very considerable. It is certainly possible to make a stimulating general review of the subject or to explain in an interesting way some recent work done in the laboratories from which the visitor is truant. But it is also possible to confuse, irritate, or bore the audience to distraction. Almost as frequent as the incomprehensible lecturer is the one who appears to consider his audience to be composed of secondary school pupils learning about the wonders of science. Another type is the rare one who has genuinely been taken by surprise, and prevailed upon to give a talk without the opportunity for adequate preparation. Unless he is supremely gifted, such talks tend to degenerate into a string of anecdotes and personal reminiscences. If the visitor is not well known locally, it is difficult to predict beforehand the category into which his discourse will fall and thus difficult to know whether or not to recommend it to students.

One unfortunate result of the proliferation of such lectures is that many student societies are on the brink of failure through lack of support; there is too much talk going on during the day for their members to wish to listen to more in the evening. It is possibly significant that the pattern of student society activities is changing. Fifty years ago talks and discussions were provided very largely by the students themselves, but currently their meetings are addressed mostly by local medical graduates or by visitors, and the tradition of student speakers is dying. Nevertheless it is excellent training for a student to work up a subject to the point where he can give a lecture on it to his fellows, and many departments still require this from their charges, although the great increase of student numbers renders it much more difficult to organize.

Like sermons, lectures have become shorter. In the old days it was not uncommon for a lecturer to go on for $1\frac{1}{2}$ hours, and I myself have sat through some sessions of 2 hours' duration. Nowadays it is generally held that no lecture should go on for more than 45 minutes, but many lecturers still occupy the full hour which became traditional in the early part of this century. It is just as absurd to insist that no lecture should last more than 45 minutes as it is to insist that no lecture should last less than 1 hour, for all the scientific work on attention spans and mental fatigue does not, and cannot, make allowance for the differing skills of the lecturer and for the intrinsic interest of the subject for the particular audience. With some lecturers an hour passes very quickly and happily; with others 10 minutes is too long. But if the whole hour which the timetable provides is occupied in one-sided exposition, there is no time left for the students to take part in a discussion afterwards. This defect can be remedied by the provision of seminars [see p. 108].

It is now common to issue the class with synopses of what the lecturer has said or is going to say. This can be carried to undesirable extremes, for the synopses are sometimes so full as to constitute a transcript of the lecture, thus relieving the student at one stroke of any need to attend the lecture or to attempt to think for himself. Lecturing is not an entertainment laid on by lecturers for the benefit of a passive audience, but a combined effort which ought to be contributed to by all those present. It is just as difficult and responsible a task to listen to a lecture as it is to give one, and to issue detailed sheets of this kind is to deprive the student of most of what makes lectures valuable, and to substitute yet another (and often inferior) supply of reading material.

Opponents of lectures often argue that it is unfair to compel a student to attend lectures, and so to provide a captive audience for second-rate performances. But in most medical schools lectures are no longer compulsory, and the spectacle of the professor standing with the nominal roll in his hand, checking off each student as he comes in, has long vanished from the scene.

It is often difficult to decide who should give the lectures. In Scotland, in the preclinical departments, the introductory lectures are frequently given by the most senior member of staff available (*Hale Report*, 1964). It is, of course, self-evident to anyone who has been through a university course that the most senior member of the departmental teaching staff is not necessarily the one who can lecture best. But he has usually had enough experience to be able to take a wider view of his subject than the juniors, whose minds are often cluttered up with the detail necessary for the acquisition of higher degrees or postgraduate professional diplomas. His lectures are therefore less likely to be full of paralysing detail.

If at all possible, the best lecturer that the department can command should be selected for the early stages, when the students have difficulty in comprehending what the subject is all about; those who are not so adept should be reserved for the later stages when the students have some sort of background against which they can measure, and into which they can fit, the new knowledge which is being presented. It may be desirable for the most skilful lecturer on the staff to appear again at the end of the course, in an attempt to summarize briefly the material which has been given throughout the year. This, like the comparable task of summarizing the contributions to a symposium, is a formidable assignment, and is not always very well done.

I believe, with Marshall (1969*a*), that in the medical curriculum lectures have a particular place which cannot easily be taken over by anything else. Small group teaching may exercise the student's brain more than lectures, but given a stimulating lecturer (and it is a big proviso) lectures are always the most economical and least time-consuming, and also often the best, method of presenting a topic. It is for this reason that they have survived the attacks which have been made on them in the last 20 years, and are still entrenched in most medical schools. There is, indeed, a considerable danger that the unthinking adoption of such slogans as 'Cut down lectures' may actually damage the standard of teaching in some departments, while only marginally improving it in others.

Small Group Teaching

Quite apart from the merits or demerits of lectures as such, but exercising an incalculable influence on their survival, is the difficulty —in some cases the impossibility—of replacing them by other methods of verbal communication. It is hardly sensible that as attempts are being made to reduce the size of classes in primary schools on the grounds that large classes mean bad teaching, considerable increases in the size of classes at the universities should be enforced for purely financial reasons. Confronted by a class of 150 or more, which is currently said to represent the economic minimum for survival of the institution (*Report of the Royal Commission*, 1968), the faculty of medicine looks round despairingly for sufficient staff to man the tutorials, the seminars, and the debates which the reformers urge upon them. All these methods are far more expensive of teaching effort than lectures, and, particularly in the preclinical departments, suitably qualified staff are now so thin upon the ground that their very replacement is a matter for anxiety, let alone their proliferation. Very few medical graduates are nowadays prepared to allow their enthusiasm for human biology to blind them to the economic facts of life [see p. 43], and for many preclinical departments such small group teaching as they may be able to mount is in consequence done almost exclusively by junior science graduates.

In the clinical departments most of the staff have medical degrees, but they face the ever-present problem of clinical care. It is much easier to give one lecture to the class than to meet small segments of it perhaps eight or nine times to repeat the same material, and clinical small group teachers often wear the aspect of the hunted fawn during term-time. Since teaching of this kind goes on throughout most of the year, it is not perhaps surprising that so many clinical teachers forget their seminars, and do not turn up to play their part in important combined teaching sessions.

The principle of teaching in small groups stems from the tutorial system of Oxford and Cambridge, in which each student is allotted to a tutor who sees him once a week to discuss his problems, examine his progress, and stimulate his endeavours, as well as to supervise his reading and to stress the essential points in it. Such an expensive system is obviously very difficult to institute in large faculties of medicine, and even at Oxford tutorials are now often given in small groups rather than individually. (The *Hale Report* arbitrarily defines tutorials as discussions in which no more than four students take part; a discussion group larger than this is called a seminar. Although the words are often used interchangeably, most discussion groups in the faculty of medicine are by this definition seminars. The tutorial is, as the *Hale Report* indicates, student-centred, the teacher being concerned mainly with the individual problems of the students concerned, while the seminar is subject-centred, the teacher being concerned primarily to secure adequate understanding and discussion of a given topic.)

Most teachers would agree that small group teaching is the ideal way of establishing contact with the individual student and his difficulties, of allowing him to obtain information suited to his own particular problems, and of making him feel that he is not simply a unit in a card index, but someone in whom the faculty has a personal interest. Nevertheless, the system is not free from objections.

Small group instruction is more demanding than a course of lectures, because it requires greater active co-operation from the students. This may be very difficult in the early stages of the curriculum, at a time when the students are very self-conscious, and do not know each other very well. Those who are capable of adequate co-operation often do not wish to provide it, for fear of being thought different from the others. There may be special difficulties in Scotland, where some students may never have used their own minds before, and have certainly never been called upon to do so in public. It is also a sad commentary on the relationship between teachers and schoolchildren that the common attitude of many students is one of distrust. It is thought to be better to keep one's mouth shut and be thought a fool than to open it and prove it. Tutors in the first few years of the curriculum therefore have to spend a good deal of time in gaining confidence. The suspicion with which they are regarded may take a year or so to overcome, and during this time the small group sessions are inefficient because the students take a minimal part in them.[2] Later on, the more adult product handed on to the clinicians may derive considerable benefit from small group sessions.

Part of the difficulty may almost be called iatrogenic, since it stems from another remedial reform, this time of the examination system. The concepts of intercurrent and continuous assessment [see p. 145], which students claim to welcome, sometimes induce those of a suspicious or paranoid turn of mind to feel that in their small groups they are more vulnerable to being spied upon, and that every word they say is probably written down in a little book by the tutor, to be used in evidence.

In small groups of students it is easy to detect enthusiasm, slacking, dullness, co-operation, and originality. The discussion group is not, as the *Hale Report* indicates, suitable for logical exposition, and tends to become incoherent and digressive. In groups of mixed attainments it often happens that progress is made at the pace of the slowest member present, and it is seldom that advances in knowledge can be as thoroughly presented as in a suitable lecture, for the essence

---

[2] As the Hale committee points out, because a student is unresponsive to this kind of teaching it does not follow that he does not need it; his very unresponsiveness may be a sign of his need.

of teaching of this kind is its spontaneity. Many tutors find this difficult, and may as a result convert their small group teaching into a series of 'mini-lectures'—a device which nullifies the whole concept.

Students say they enjoy tutorials and seminars more than other forms of teaching, and rank them fairly highly in terms of value (*Report of the Royal Commission*, 1968), though one might not think so from the general demeanour of the actual participants when asked to make a contribution. Teachers also enjoy them, for they afford them an opportunity for getting to know one small segment of the class in much greater detail than it is ever possible to know the whole class. This again carries with it its own dangers, for there is more scope for personal antagonisms to be aroused in a small group of people. This can to a certain extent be avoided if the student group rotates among a series of different tutors during their course. In this way each tutor gets to know a substantial number of the class, and at the same time each student has the opportunity of profiting by the various teaching styles and personal experiences of several different people. The drawback to this system is that it fails to achieve the rapport which can grow between a tutor and his flock if he is in charge of them for a longer period.

In the classical tutorial system of the ancient universities the medical faculty has more problems than other faculties. This is because of the multiplicity of different subjects involved. If a student is reading, say, economics, it is quite possible for a single tutor to supervise his studies throughout his entire course, for the number of subjects studied is relatively small, and they are taken to a reasonable depth. In the medical faculty, however, it is rare for any one tutor to be able to cope satisfactorily with more than a limited range of subjects. Thus, if the tutor is a pharmacologist, he may not be able to help the student with his surgical difficulties, and if he is a bio-chemist, he may have little skill in dealing with pathological problems. For this reason several tutors are necessary to cover the range of medical subjects, and each one has to gain the student's confidence. This takes time, and detracts from the value of the system.

It is really only in departments where the students spend a considerable slice of their education that the small group system comes into full flower. But departments in which the student does not have a long stay can use seminars in a 'subject-centred' manner [see p. 108] —to demonstrate a point which would otherwise be difficult for the individual to see or understand, to discuss a particularly confusing aspect of the subject, or to place before the group certain advances in technique or in knowledge. These sessions are often really demonstrations rather than small group teaching as it is generally understood. For example, in the department of diagnostic radiology students usually watch screening sessions in small groups, unless television is available on a big scale.

Clinical seminars present another difficulty. To ensure a fair assessment of student performance, it is desirable that each small group should have a series of similar clinical experiences. But the hospital does not always contain a sufficient number of patients with very similar clinical signs and symptoms, and even the most co-operative patient eventually resents being used over and over again for teaching purposes. The result is that each group sees a different series of patients, and important clinical conditions may be omitted from the experience of one group, but not from that of others. This difficulty can be partly met by giving an initial presentation to the whole class, after which it breaks up into small sections. Each section tutor knows beforehand what had been said at the initial presentation, and can thus select a series of clinical cases bearing directly on this material. If this sort of thing is not done, the clinical experience of some groups of students may be wholly uncoordinated with the formal course of lectures [see p. 88], and it is a common defect of the clinical teaching system in this country that there is a lack of communication between those responsible for the lecture courses and those responsible for the tutorials and clinical demonstrations.

In Oxford a clinical tutorial system, staffed from the academic departments and from the ranks of the registrars and consultants, and similar in most respects to the classical Oxford system, has been in operation since 1948. Another such scheme started after the war in the London Hospital (Ellis, 1956b). Badenoch (1967), discussing the Oxford scheme, makes the point that some students do not respond well to it, and that it may degenerate into 'an expensive form of personal coaching' unless the greatest care is taken to prevent this. On the other hand, feedback from the majority of students is strongly in favour of the system.

In summary, small group teaching is not always easy, either to organize or to take part in (Beard, 1970). Although a few experiments have been done to investigate its effectiveness when compared to other forms of teaching (Joyce and Weatherall, 1957; Walton, 1966) a large-scale investigation still has to be undertaken. Meanwhile it is practised with varying degrees of enthusiasm depending on the age, physical endurance, and degree of extroversion of the staff.

Combined Discussions

This type of teaching, which originated in America, is also expensive in terms of staff effort, for it involves bringing together several teachers to discuss some point which cuts across departmental boundaries. Such sessions are therefore usually tied up with the concept of integrated teaching [see p. 81]. They are difficult to organize, since they depend upon appropriate representatives from a number of departments converging on the same place at the same time, and also upon these representatives being adequately informed of the nature and purpose of the proceedings. Neither prerequisite can be guaranteed in advance.

The type specimen of such sessions is the clinicopathological conference, which, if well done, is both exciting, informative, and stimulating (Sinclair, 1955). But a great deal of hard work lies behind a successful discussion of this nature, and if the participants are inadequately briefed and unrehearsed the format of the occasion is no protection against dullness and boredom.

By its nature the CPC allows of audience participation; the parallel concept of 'topic teaching' does not always do so. In this form of verbal communication several teachers whose interests impinge on a particular topic are gathered together to form a kind of 'brains trust' in which each makes a short contribution on the subject; after these are complete the matter is thrown open for debate. The difficulty here is that few people accept the key word 'short'; many are anxious to impress the audience with the importance of their own contribution, and so exceed their time; others are anxious to score off their colleagues in debate. In either case audience participation may be minimal. The success of such occasions largely depends on adequate preparation and rehearsal (which they seldom get) and on the presence of a tall and formidable chairman like the late Sir Frederic Bartlett, who used to bend double, creep round the front of the lecture bench, and then rear up between the audience and the recalcitrant speaker who would not stop talking. A discussion must be a discussion or it fails in its purpose.

Tape-recorders

For many years the tape-recorder has been used in postgraduate medicine as a means of allowing groups of doctors in widely separated areas to obtain at least some benefit from an address given at one particular point; the tape is circulated round the various groups and perhaps eventually stored for record purposes. It has also been used in undergraduate teaching to record a particularly effective lecture for future use. But nowadays the tape-recorder is invading a new territory—that of the self-service demonstration. The technique of providing a recorded commentary on a visual display is familiar in art galleries; it is now being extended to pathological museums. Other uses include the provision of tapes in conjunction with slide-projectors to allow several students at a time to revise their normal or pathological histology, or to extend their knowledge of unfamiliar histological techniques (Fletcher and Watson, 1968). It may also be used in connexion with student-operated filmstrips or special clinical demonstrations, and the University of Newcastle upon Tyne has a collection of tape/slide presentations suitable for revision study by final-year clinical students (Amos *et al.*, 1969).

The great advantage of such techniques is that they allow individual students to proceed at their own pace and to obtain information without the presiding staff member having to be continuously present. Their disadvantage is that the recorded commentary may be inadequate, that the student cannot ask the questions which occur to him, and that the whole atmosphere is much less personal and more mechanical. But there is no doubt that, as a device for freeing staff for other duties, they have an important part to play in the coming days of staff shortage.

Listening

Most medical students arrive at the university very deficient in the art of listening. In these days, when so many children spend their evenings either watching the television while conducting a conversation with their friends, or doing their homework with the transistor radio screwed into one ear, the idea of devoting their undivided attention to the matter in hand is quite a strange one, and this is a skill which requires progressive development as the student proceeds through his medical course. Not all university teachers are equally good at commanding attention, and the student must remain alert and critical, receptive and interested. Most teachers have had the rather depressing experience of being asked, following a lecture, to explain a factual point which was stressed two or three times during the lecture itself, and every teacher has certainly found himself passing round a tutorial group with a question which has to be repeated a couple of times because the next victim was not expecting to have to answer it and had therefore shut off his mind at source. People find it easy to listen to what they themselves say, but much more difficult to listen properly to the views of others. Yet one of the fundamental necessities in clinical practice is the ability to listen critically and attentively to the stories told by patients, for in what they say very frequently lies the whole diagnosis.

THE WRITTEN WORD

Books

So much attention is nowadays being paid to new and improved teaching methods that it is sometimes forgotten that the printed word continues to be the main source of information for medical students (Sinclair, 1956b). If entirely suitable textbooks could be provided for every phase of the medical curriculum, a great deal of worry and difficulty would be avoided, for much of the effort put into educating students is directed towards overcoming the deficiencies, real or imagined, of the available reading material. Lectures are painstakingly devised to correct the errors of fact and the heretical opinions to be found in the recommended books; tutorials are arranged to illuminate the obscurities left by the author's style; sheaves of notes are distributed to fill the gaps in the author's presentation. So striking are the deficiencies of even the best textbook that the head of the department can find, that it is not surprising that most of them eventually give up the search and determine to write one themselves.

Enormous works of reference, such as were formerly recommended, find no place in modern medical curricula. If the total time available for the teaching of a particular subject is 10 hours, then it is obviously useless to recommend a three-volume textbook. But any book which is too large for its purpose is unsuitable; the students may be advised to omit certain chapters, but this is an unsatisfactory expedient. A good student feels obliged to learn it all, and a bad student, like Bluebeard's wife, finds that all the interesting bits seem to be in the forbidden portions.

Conversely, too small a book often induces a feeling of frustration in the better students, who feel that they would like to know more about the subject than they are permitted to read. The small 'cram' books, which are so popular with students round about examination time, may help them to pass the unsatisfactory 'factual' type of examination [see p. 153], but they are too brief, too didactic, and too incomplete to communicate a proper understanding of the subject. Occasionally such books are recommended, with the proviso that certain other reading is necessary. This proviso is often not followed since the student equates the 'set book' with the examination.

The expense of the medical course sets a ceiling to the number of books bought, and very few students are keen enough to spend their limited time in reading around their subjects; they therefore confine themselves for the most part to the recommended texts. It follows that most students are, as far as their reading goes, indoctrinated with only one particular viewpoint, and this means that the selection of a text is a most important matter. Most schools tend to exclude from their book list those books which have an original slant, and rely instead on solid orthodox texts with a reliable party line. This may make for safety, but it also tends towards dullness, and the best students fail to obtain the stimulation which a rather more enterprising account might provide.

The common solution to such problems is to provide in the library a series of supplementary books which the better students can be encouraged to consult. But such is the dominance of the examination system that few students actually do this. Instead they tend to complain that the library does not carry enough copies of the recommended texts. Possibly because of their price, most students are unwilling to buy books on any subject which occupies less than 200 or 300 hours in the curriculum. They prefer to borrow the set books on minor subjects from the library, or even, in extreme cases, to steal them from the library or bookshop. The curious attitude that this is not really stealing is said to derive from a belief that the State has an obligation to provide tertiary education, and also to provide every conceivable means, including books, whereby this education can be completed. If it does not do so for nothing, then taking books is justified. This convenient delusion is still rather less common in students of medicine than in students of the arts and the social sciences, and difficulties over books in the medical library are usually confined to people failing to return books when requested to do so; however, losses by stealing increase every year.

A major factor determining the reluctance of students to buy books is of course their price, and at a time when consultants are complaining (Pyke, 1969; Havard, 1969) about the high, and rising, price of medical books, it is possible to sympathize with the predicament of a student who cannot afford all the recommended books. Nevertheless, as Greene (1969) has pointed out, a large number of students hold special grants for buying books, and many actually use them. Again, many student texts are now published in an alternative paperback version, which allows some reduction in price.

Two of the most important points to be considered when selecting a book for the reading list are its clarity and its level of presentation. To arrive at a satisfactory decision the teacher must achieve the almost impossible feat of putting himself in the place of a student beginning the study of the subject. Often he does not have the time to read through the book completely, and even if he does so, he may fail to appreciate how difficult the class may find the treatment of a particular topic, which to him is perfectly clear because of his previous knowledge. The standard of production of medical textbooks is nowadays extremely good, and profuse illustrations cater splendidly for the visual memory; it is the text which often falls short of perfection. It was once unkindly said that there are two kinds of lectures—lectures with pictures and lectures with thoughts. The same comment can sometimes be applied to books, and the student whose memory and understanding are stimulated better by words than by pictures may sometimes be at a disadvantage. The Chinese proverb that a little picture is worth a thousand words may be true for some topics, but it is equally true that it is difficult or impossible to embody principles and abstract thought in illustrations: how, for example, does one illustrate the Golden Rule? On the other hand many texts, though full of irreproachable facts and sentiments, are almost unreadable, because the author paid insufficient attention to writing simply and clearly (Sinclair, 1956*b*).

A curious point relating to books arises in conjunction with combined or integrated courses of instruction [see p. 81]. Some teachers feel that such courses should not be given until a suitable textbook is available. Thus, should the department of anatomy and the department of radiology combine together to give a course of microradiology, the argument is that this course should be postponed until a suitable elementary textbook of microradiology for medical students is available. This argument would convert such courses into simply additional 'subjects', with their own lectures, tutorials, textbooks, and (inevitably) departments and professors. This is merely adding to the curriculum instead of introducing a new form of educative process—integration has always been something which the student must do in his own mind or it loses its value. Nevertheless, books which attempt to integrate or combine the work of many individual departments are now appearing, and a satisfactory integrated text for each phase of the curriculum would undoubtedly help both students and staff.[3]

It is also only a question of time before programmed texts for medical students make their appearance. Already such texts exist in medical subjects for the use of nurses, radiographers, and other paramedical workers, and some attempts have been made to cover such topics as electrocardiography (Owen, 1966) by this technique. However, there are formidable difficulties about adopting them in the medical curriculum. In the first place, to present anything more than a very simple coverage of the subject in this format makes the book very large, and in morphological subjects there may be difficulty over the illustrations. Secondly, there is trouble over the baseline of knowledge to be assumed. In programming a text of (say) pathology the programmer should know what was taught in previous years of the curriculum; if he starts from zero knowledge, the first part of the text is insufferably elementary and tedious. Yet the content of the courses preceding that of pathology is so diverse in different places that a programmed text of this kind might have a very limited appeal. Thirdly, the technique of 'true or false' or 'fill-in' questions which most of these books use is ill-adapted to medical subjects, where most questions have answers which are neither confidently black nor assuredly white, but rather uncertainly grey. In mathematics or technology programming may be quite satisfactory, but no sooner does one have to answer any question in biology or medicine with one word or phrase than one begins to wish to qualify the answer, and the better the student the more he feels this need [see p. 149]. To deny him the opportunity, and to imply that every problem in a given subject can be satisfactorily answered by the insertion of one from a selection of words provided for him, is to give him a most unsatisfactory background for his future life's work. Finally, the techniques of programming either a book or a machine do not yet rest on a perfectly secure foundation and some of the methods adopted may actually produce confusion in the student's mind (Biran and Pickering, 1968).

Reading

Reading is a habit which is nowadays much more difficult to acquire than it used to be. Most students have stuck to the 'set' books

[3] Malleson (1968) suggests that if a modular form of curriculum should be adopted, a new type of book could be needed, in which the material could be continuously serviced by a looseleaf system. Such books would include at intervals a self-assessment programme, lists of material such as museum specimens to be studied, and references to original work appropriate to that part of the course.

required of them at school, a procedure which may well get them through examinations but gives them no claim to be educated. The suggestion that medical students should read widely and try to get some general background, is always greeted with the defensive reaction that 'there isn't time'. If this defence is examined carefully, it transpires that most of their time in the evenings is spent in conversation with other students, watching television, playing billiards, going to the cinema, drinking beer—almost anything, in fact, except reading. Dr. Johnson once said, 'A man ought to read just as inclination leads him, for what he reads as a task will do him little good'. This is impossible advice for a medical student to follow, but if he concentrates only on the technical literature of his trade he will miss one of the greatest pleasures of life. Too many people qualify in medicine in ignorance of most of the glorious span of English literature from Jane Austen to space fiction. Those who do not make time for reading during their student days seldom take it after qualification, and it is they who justify the criticism that the medical profession is often narrow-minded. This is not an argument for compulsory courses of 'culture' [see p. 96] in the curriculum, but merely a suggestion that reading in one's spare time is still a worthwhile form of activity and a guarantee against a lonely and cantankerous old age.

Many students at the time of entry to the medical school have not acquired the very necessary habit of *critical* reading, for they have failed to appreciate that textbooks are written by fallible and prejudiced human beings. They have to shed their superstitious reverence for the printed word and to get rid of the idea that 'it must be true, it's in the book' [see p. 24]. They have to learn that the quick skim through which suffices to disclose the plot of a thriller is totally inadequate to unravel the secrets of pathology or genetics; they have, in fact, to learn the distinction between reading for business and reading for pleasure or to pass the time away.

Although the ASME survey (*Report of the Royal Commission*, 1968) reveals that final-year students rate the reading of textbooks very highly as a means of learning, students in earlier years have often not learned how to get the best out of their books (Sinclair, 1956*b*). They have to be told that in the evenings they should look up the conditions they see in the wards during the day, that they should use their lecture notes and their textbooks to supplement each other, that they should stop at intervals as they read and make sure they have understood the section they have just covered. Some university *graduates* have to be told the value of an index as a means of finding one's way through an unfamiliar book (Beard, 1970). Such ideas, odd though it may seem, do not always come naturally to university students, and the pity is that nobody seems to think it necessary to give them instruction and practice in the art of reading. The brief introductory courses which so many universities nowadays give to all new students either before or in the first few days of their first university term (*Hale Report*, 1964) are almost useless for such purposes, since the newcomers find everything so strange and new that they cannot take in what is being said to them properly, let alone act upon it. It is better to issue new students with a written pamphlet summarizing such advice, for, if they do not lose it, they can refer to it later when they find themselves in trouble.

Writing

Another skill which medical students must acquire, if they do not already have it, is that of writing. The objective examination [see p. 149] has not yet completely taken over, and many of the examinations in the medical faculty still take the form of essay questions. These demand an ability to arrange facts and opinions into a connected coherent story, which must be written in English, with appropriate punctuation marks, and some rudimentary attention to grammar. Those who fail in such examinations in the early stages of the curriculum because they have no idea of how to set things down are nearly as numerous as those who fail through lack of knowledge, for one of the major problems in most universities today is that students cannot adequately communicate. It is therefore essential that they should be taught to say exactly what they mean, clearly, completely, and concisely. It was Pascal who apologized for writing a friend such a long letter, because he had not had the time to write him a short one. Taking notes at the bedside or in the clinic is an admirable way of learning how to set down the essentials of the matter without any flowery verbiage.

To require students to write essays has been a recognized way of inducing them to learn something about a subject since the early days of the Oxford and Cambridge tutorial system. Under this regime the student writes an essay on a set subject, and this is then discussed and individually criticized by the tutor, after which it may be modified, and perhaps rewritten. Like most educational methods, this one stands or falls by the human element. Writing essays can soon degenerate into a mechanical chore in which received opinion from textbooks is padded out with information from a rather more dashing article discovered in the library, supplemented with the latest thing from the television science programmes. The student learns nothing except how to copy things out in a paraphrased version.

On the other hand, should the essay be cunningly set, things are different. The usual sources of information may reveal little in the way of essay-fodder, and the necessity for filling a reasonable space with words may actually drive the student inside his own skull to ferret there for opinions he is sometimes startled to realize he possesses. If the tutor insists on proper presentation and meaningful English instead of dreary jargon, the whole exercise may come to life and the essay system may provide the most valuable lessons the student learns during the whole of his course.

But how easily the method, excellent in itself, is abused! In some departments essays are regularly required of the whole class. At first they are handed in with some apprehension, tinged perhaps with excitement. But as the weeks go by and the essays are neither returned nor discussed, these emotions undergo an inevitable slackening, and a list of bare marks, put up on the board without comment, does little to restore morale. When the next essay is asked for, many students have found out that the same essays were set 3 years ago, and that some senior students still have copies of the ones they wrote (and occasionally received good marks for). The more daring act accordingly, and when no thunderbolts fall from heaven the whole system is thoroughly discredited.

It is very difficult for the staff to maintain interest in a whole batch of student essays, some of which are inevitably extremely jejune. The marking is therefore often entrusted to juniors, who, themselves educated in the 'look and say' method at school, may be fairly uncertain of their own command of the English language.[4] As a consequence students may get very little out of the essay system, either in terms of expression or in terms of information, and they may even acquire a lasting disinclination towards writing anything down.

Arithmetic

The third 'R' of university education is the one with which medical students tend to have most difficulty, for few of them are by nature numerate [see p. 130]. But now that so much research and so many medical publications are based on statistics, it is essential that medical students should understand the basic statistical ideas and methods,

---

[4] Hubble (1960) tells the story of the scientific visitor to Harwell who, when asked to sign his name, put two crosses in the visitors' book. 'What is the second cross for?', asked the receptionist. 'That's my Ph.D.' was the proud reply.

and indeed instruction in biometric methods is firmly recommended by the General Medical Council (1967). Most courses in statistics include a few examples, for, in statistics as in all other subjects, principles are easier to understand if clothed in facts, or, in this case, figures. The emphasis placed on actual working of examples varies, but in many courses there are 'example classes' which are an excellent source of 'feedback' on the material included in the lectures (*Hale Report*, 1964). Students may be given the opportunity of machine calculations, and may have a demonstration of computer operation.

The main difficulty is to make them take such procedures seriously, and the best solution is probably for each of the other departments in the medical course to make a point of stressing the statistical aspects of their subjects (Sinclair, 1955). In the student's inexperienced eyes the mathematics taught by a mathematician is often regarded as a piece of useless 'frightfulness'. But if he sees this mathematics in daily use by medical workers he may be induced to change his view and to attempt to acquire a vitally useful mode of thought.

THE PICTURES

Some lecturers still adhere to the 'chalk and talk' school of thought, but others, particularly the younger ones, use all kinds of visual aids and appurtenances. To the non-mechanically minded, the lecture bench of many theatres resembles the control room of a power station; overhead projectors lurk at its edges, knobs and switches abound, and little dials display the time, the humidity, and the state of affairs in the projection room. With a touch batteries of projectors can be brought into simultaneous play, the lights can be dimmed, the windows closed, or (and more likely) the fuses blown.

Those who adopt the trendy approach to lecturing put constant pressure on the reactionaries to invest in some electrons and enter the space age. When it is pointed out that Socrates had no need of power-operated blackboards, or of closed-circuit television, they reply that if he were alive today he would be the first to ask the Vice-Chancellor to obtain them. Alas, most such appliances are expensive, and in the present financial climate they are luxuries, which all Vice-Chancellors are conditioned to resist.

Apart from the need for amplification systems, most of the devices

IBE

which embroider modern medical teaching are products of the belief that no form of teaching is meaningful without adequate visual illustration. No lecture is thus complete without its cargo of slides, and every lecture theatre must have at least two motion picture projectors, one for 35 mm and another for 16 mm films. If it is to be in the technical swim, it must also have television facilities, or, better still, a complete television system of its own.

Blackboard and Overhead Projector

It may seem strange to begin with a method of illustration which nowadays attracts no attention whatsoever. The days of the master blackboard illustrators are over, precisely because of the excellence of more modern and less difficult methods of illustration. Yet blackboard *diagrams* still have an extremely important—not to say basic—role to play in medical illustration. They are easy to produce and for the student to copy, they can be built up step by step in front of the class, and they still command more attention than the evanescent stimulus of a transparency which is whisked on and off and which the student gets no time to copy (Barabas, 1965). It is essential that blackboard drawings should be kept as simple as possible, and that too much detail should be avoided. The value of the drawing lies in its immediacy and in the fact that the student gains in understanding by reproducing it—if it is too complicated this objective is defeated, and there are nearly always much better pictures in the textbook.

The overhead projector has similar potentialities, and allows the speaker to remain facing the class while drawing. It has the additional advantage that it can be used to display radiographs or other transparent material previously prepared without the necessity of switching to another instrument. But this very advantage may induce the lecturer to prepare complicated drawings beforehand and so lose much of the value of the technique.

Transparencies

For many years the medical illustration departments of various medical faculties throughout Britain have been reporting a steady increase in work load, the bulk of which represents the demand for 35 mm transparencies. Most of those provided by them are filed away in a dark cupboard in the recipient's room in the delusion that they will be needed at some unspecified time in the future, but a substantial proportion are actually shown to other people, either at a scientific meeting or in a lecture to undergraduates. In both cases it is usual to find that half a dozen transparencies are used where one would prove just as impressive and a great deal less boring. This is particularly the case when the transparencies show microscopic preparations, either from the light or from the electron microscope.

The quality of transparencies is very variable—not, if they are made by experts, in technical excellence, but in educational impact. Despite several useful articles on the subject (e.g. Williams, 1965), many teachers intent on presenting technical data still insist on cramming the frame full of too much numerical information, so that it becomes actively confusing, and it ought to be the job of the medical illustration department to restrain them. At the other extreme are the transparencies insisted upon by senior clinicians giving postgraduate lectures, in which perhaps five words carefully typewritten in yellow on a brilliant blue background appear momentarily, to be replaced by further sets of five words in rapid succession. Usually they read out the words slowly in case anybody missed them.

On the other hand, excellent transparencies can be made of clinical conditions and these are of inestimable value in illustrating verbal descriptions. It is this basic distinction between what is or is not visual *by its nature* that is lacking in many teachers' minds.

Film and Filmstrip

The teaching film is often a dangerous weapon, since so few are satisfying. The idea behind showing a film is to enable the whole class to see a method, a disease process, or an unusual clinical condition, with a minimum of trouble to themselves and to other people. This is a laudable objective, but few scientists are also expert film-makers, and many medical films are still made which induce, not interest and the 'ah-ha' reaction, but boredom and even hilarity. It is always difficult to restain film-makers from prolixity, and a good editor is even more important in educational than in commercial film-making. Many films are made which ignore the basic premise that the duty of a moving picture is to move, and show nothing more than what could perfectly well be shown at a fraction of the cost by means of colour transparencies (Marshall, 1953).

A film is of course impersonal, and people have been immunized against experiences of this kind by the cinema and television, so that their minds and bodies erect defences against the assault on their senses. A student who has been accustomed to sit in front of the family television playing cards with one eye on the programme finds

it difficult to swivel his mind around to confront the material presented squarely, and with comprehension as well as attention. The
darkness induces a pleasurable hypnotic effect, enhanced by the
background music which most film-makers consider indispensable;
the critical faculty is suspended, and those who call for a discussion
among the audience about the fascinating exposition they have just
had the pleasure of watching are usually disappointed.

Nevertheless some admirable medical films exist, and there is no
question that if a student ought to see something which cannot be
presented to him in solid and concrete form a film can be an excellent
way of giving him the experience (Claxton and Quilliam, 1968).

Filmstrip is profitably used to demonstrate short techniques, or
processes which are quickly over and are difficult to follow at a single
viewing, for they have the advantage of allowing endless repetition.
Such matters as the course of events in a barium swallow afford an
ideal example. Some departments make filmstrips available to students
on a self-service basis in the museum or practical classroom, and the
strip may be hooked up to an explanatory tape-recorder [see p. 113].

One field in which one would expect film to be extremely effective
is in the teaching of embryology by means of cartoon techniques. But
although a beginning has been made[5] very little has as yet been done
in this direction, in which films would seem to have an overwhelming
advantage over static diagrams and books.

Television and Videotape

Television teaching sometimes suffers from a disability common to
many operations in which electrons are engaged, that the method
tends to replace the objectives. This is perhaps best demonstrated by
hi-fi enthusiasts, who may spend years building a machine to give
perfect sound reproduction, and then lose interest once it has been
completed, so that they never actually *use* it for anything.

In the initial stages of enthusiasm for television, large sums of
money were spent on the assumption that this was the answer to
teaching large classes. It is indeed possible to use it in this way, for
example to accommodate overflow audiences when a visiting lecturer
gives a popular talk, but such arrangements are seldom as satisfactory
as seeing the lecturer in the flesh.

---

[5] For example, W. J. Hamilton, J. D. Boyd, and T. W. Glenister, in conjunction with
Messrs. Macmillan and Orriss Animations Ltd., have produced a series of 8mm cartoon
filmstrips on the development of the oocyte, fertilization, and the early stages of
development of the blastocyst.

Television can also be used for demonstrating fine structural details. It may therefore find a place in histology classes, where time may be saved by the demonstrator if he can display the section which the class is studying and go over its details with the whole class at once, instead of going round to assist each individual student (Olson, 1970). But a good series of colour transparencies is just about as effective, and unbelievably cheaper. Another application of television is in osteology classes or pathology demonstrations. The difficulties of showing a whole class the foramina on the base of a normal-sized skull are sufficiently obvious, but if an enlarged image of the bone can be projected on to a number of screens, they are much reduced (Meyrick, 1968). However, the modern lack of emphasis on anatomical detail has rendered this kind of usage less important. The drawbacks of television teaching in preclinical practical classes have been well summarized by Olson (1970). Apart from the cost, they include technical problems in regard to siting of the monitors, the possibility of technical failures during teaching, 'hypnosis' of the recipients, magnification of faults in presentation, and limitation, not only of the type of information which can be conveyed, but also of the amount which can be tolerated at any one time.

Experiments have been made in the teaching of surgery in a 'television clinic' (Smith and Wyllie, 1965; Smith, Wyllie, Foote, and Caridis, 1966) and in the teaching of neurology (Cantrell and Craven, 1969). But perhaps the most useful place for television is in the operating theatre, where the details of an operative procedure can be displayed to many people at once. This requirement is also less needed than formerly in the undergraduate curriculum, and in general the application of television in undergraduate teaching is less certain than it was some years ago; it is finding a bigger role in the postgraduate phase of medical education.

In both phases the chief difficulty is one of expense. To be of maximal value for clinical purposes, the television should be in colour, and this adds greatly to the cost. Live transmissions from the ward or operating theatre to various places in the hospital—lecture theatres, classrooms and so on—necessitate expensive land-lines, and lead to the provision of a central studio where the technical facilities necessary for the operation of the system can be more efficiently grouped and operated. Such a studio in turn requires staff, and so the empire grows. Many places have in fact given up the idea of having live transmissions at all, and rely on the use of videotape for teaching.

Videotape is the latest fashion. Many medical schools have already invested much capital in apparatus for the production and viewing of such tapes, and they are claimed to have certain advantages. For example, they are said to be excellent for recording a physiological experiment which is difficult to repeat or prepare; the tape can be run over and over again, and many people can view at the same time. Videotape is particularly suitable for demonstrating functional radiography—the movements of joints, the screening of a barium series, and so on (Davidson and Thomson, 1970). It can be used to display the features of an interesting clinical case, and other uses will spring to mind, But it is difficult to appreciate just why videotape, which is very expensive and difficult to organize, should be much superior to a well-produced film. Videotape in colour is too expensive for routine use, and black and white tape loses both colour and the immediacy which is the chief value of live television. If the same expenditure were to be allotted to the production of medical films by professional film producers as is at present being allotted to the production of television programmes and videotape by television producers, there would appear to be no reason why film should not be just as satisfactory (Brooke, 1970). No doubt videotape will extend its usefulness as the cost of production falls, and will probably come to establish a place in medical teaching which complements rather than supplants the use of film (Quilliam, 1968).

Teaching Machines

Another development making use of electrons is the use of teaching machines, though this is as yet limited (Jason, 1968). The argument runs that the teaching machine is able to adjust itself to the progress of the student, whereas in a normal teaching class the pace is too slow for the most gifted and too fast for the slowest of the students present. With a teaching machine the victim is in control of the situation and can re-run the question and answer session if he is not sure of any point. But the whole method depends on the programming, and if this is inadequate or slipshod, the procedure falls to the ground. Programming a teaching machine is a job for an expert, and very few experts are to be found in the medical faculty. For this reason teaching machines have as yet made little headway in the curriculum. Nevertheless it is possible that they have a considerable future, for curiosity and the stimulus of successful problem-solving are powerful drives which this method of learning exploits to the full (Millar, 1962).

DEMONSTRATIONS

Demonstrations are of two kinds, permanent and temporary. Brief demonstrations are often combined with lectures, and may be extremely effective, as the Christmas lectures at the Royal Institution usually exemplify. In the earliest stages of the medical curriculum chemical reactions are demonstrated to the class by means of some striking colour change or the ringing of a bell, and such occasions never fail to produce a delighted chorus of stamping or of groans. Later, in histology, class demonstrations of unusual staining methods or of comparative material are met with rather more restrained enthusiasm, and complicated physiological demonstrations (which may or may not work) are often held to be a waste of time.[6] For a class demonstration to be wholly successful, the demonstrator must be a showman of a particular kind, and not everyone can bring them off.

The former emphasis on anatomical and pathological museums is now much less evident, and many of them have been pruned of irrelevant excrescences to enable them to concentrate on the matter in hand. New methods of display are being tried out, and the museum may exhibit a 'specimen of the week' relevant to the material being taught at the time, and given the full treatment accorded to surgical demonstrations at international meetings. Copies of articles from journals may be displayed to illustrate the clinical implications of the specimens—for example, a review of the symptomatology of acute appendicitis may accompany a demonstration of the range of positions occupied by the appendix—or a tape-recording may give a commentary on the current exhibition [see p. 113].

The value of such demonstrations does not appear to have been questioned, but it is not known how much benefit students obtain from them. The theory is that they wander round them, picking up odd bits of information which do not lend themselves to oral disquisition. In some museums a system of self-instruction has been adopted (Sobin, 1968). The student is provided with a written guide to the specimens illustrating a particular anatomical system, and the flow of instruction is interrupted at intervals by questions requiring short written responses, which are handed in and assessed.

Radiological demonstrations are in use in most medical schools,

---

[6] Joyce and Weatherall (1959) found that in dealing with the pharmacology of the peripheral nervous system demonstrations were more economical than practical classes and the students enjoyed them more. There was no difference in the examination results whichever method was employed.

and are often accompanied by questions which the students can answer from observation of the films presented. There is little doubt that such demonstrations form an essential basis on which the student can build as he gains practical experience in the interpretation of radiographs.

PRACTICAL WORK

A common criticism of the orthodox curriculum has always been that it was too theoretical, and that students did not gain enough experience of the kind of things they would be expected to do once they had qualified—setting up drips, taking blood, putting on plasters, and so on. This criticism, which stems from the days of the 'safe doctor', is still heard in places like Australia, where British graduates are indeed ill-prepared for medical practice in the outback. Considering that something like 20 per cent of British graduates apparently leave this country shortly after graduation to take up practice overseas the criticism has some force. In Britain the stated objective of the curriculum is now to produce a balanced graduate who is scientifically based, and the practical attainments which are necessary to him in clinical practice are assumed to come, in large part, after he qualifies (*Report of the Royal Commission*, 1968). Nevertheless the current emphasis on 'science' as opposed to 'practice' will inevitably increase the difficulties faced by British graduates confronted by an emergency in the Australian bush or the African jungle (Thomson, 1966).

The second view of practical work is that it is a better way of learning than is attendance at lectures or other similar classes, which are thought to be essentially 'passive' [see p. 101]. This feeling is expressed in the slogan, 'Learn by doing'. At first sight this slogan is irreproachable; it is surely apparent that the best way for anyone to learn anything is to do it for himself, and the case for practical work sounds unanswerable. Nevertheless, like every such slogan, this one does not stand generalization. Practical experience is undoubtedly necessary for the acquisition of practical skills, but practical work in the curriculum at present extends far beyond this objective, and is used to further the student's theoretical knowledge in a number of ways which need close examination. The case for practical work of this kind is not nearly so clear.

Preclinical

In the preclinical part of the curriculum the chief exponent of the value of practical work is the anatomy department. It has been assumed for many years that the best way of learning the relationships of the various components of the human body is to dissect a dead body and see for oneself how the parts are arranged. The three-dimensional arrangements are very difficult to appreciate from the two-dimensional diagrams in the textbook, and models afford only a rigid and static picture of one phase of dissection. But the educative value of dissection is frequently questioned, and such experimental evidence as exists (Sinclair, 1965a) is equivocal. But at least there is an excellent reason for asking students to dissect the body, provided the basic assumption is correct. The gradual process of dissection has another, more general educational value, for it brings the class into a situation where they educate each other during the process of growing up; in no other form of practical class do such opportunities exist for discussion between student and student, or between staff and student. Another point in favour of dissection is that it allows time for the class to absorb and learn to use the immense new vocabulary on which their future studies are based. Now that so few students have even an elementary acquaintance with either Latin or Greek, it becomes more and more difficult, and more and more time-consuming, for them to pick up the language in which the business of medicine is transacted. Practical work in the dissecting room also trains the student to observe, to be careful and meticulous in the use of his hands and eyes, to develop his visual memory, and to think in three dimensions. Those who would abolish dissection altogether might, therefore, be surprised at the general effects which would follow, quite apart from the deficiencies in anatomical knowledge which would fairly certainly result.[7]

The anatomy department also makes considerable use of practical histological work, in which the student is required to learn how to use a microscope, and how to identify the tissues of the body and the way in which they are made up into organs and systems. Here again the objective is readily understood; microscopic work enters into a number of other subjects in the curriculum, and experience in it is useful to many graduates and essential to some. Examining

[7] The experience of Denmark is relevant. Between 1956 and 1967 no dissection was done because of a shortage of bodies. Because students and clinicians alike agreed that the resultant standard of anatomical understanding was not satisfactory, the anatomists were requested to reintroduce dissection as soon as cadavers could be obtained (Smart, 1971).

histological sections also contributes towards developing the student's powers of observation, and teaches him to assemble various items of data in order to come to a conclusion, as well as training him to see beyond the superficial appearances of a structure. The same applies to the practical classes in pathological histology. Yet here again caution is needed. Nowadays, few medical graduates make much use of the microscope in clinical practice, and histological diagnosis is usually done in the laboratory. The factual information derived from study of a slide in the laboratory is little superior to the factual information derived from study of a good histological atlas, for both provide merely two-dimensional pictures of a three-dimensional structure. Again, histological detail may easily get out of hand, for histologists are usually enthusiasts who desire to share their delight in the composition of pretty pictures, and the box of class slides may swell beyond the limits of the value of the method. To teach the fine distinctions between various kinds of brain tumours, for example, is of no value to the majority of students.

Other departments contributing to the preclinical curriculum also give practical classes designed to train the faculties of observation and interpretation. Physiology and pharmacology, for example, may require the student to inspect the reactions of the pupils to light and accommodation, to observe the thresholds of various forms of sensation, and to note the results of administering drugs to the intact human subject. Other experiments are given for a different reason. The blood pressures of the class may be taken, their blood counts may be examined, or their oxygen consumption recorded, in order to obtain a range of values; the main point is the variation between subjects and how this may be treated statistically. Medical students commonly appear to be deficient in the numerical sciences. This may be in part because they have specialized early at school in biology, and in part because skill in mathematics appears to accompany proficiency in the physical, rather than in the biological sciences. Yet in modern medicine it is very necessary for the student to be able to think in a numerate fashion, and practical classes of this kind are designed to help him to do so. Still other experiments are designed to bring home to the student more forcibly matters which he might otherwise simply glance over in his textbook. They therefore function largely as demonstrations.

A third group of experiments, of more questionable value, is exemplified by those in which the student may be asked to investigate a series of chemical reactions, and is given detailed instructions as to how this should be done. He may, for example, be provided with a test tube full of solution A, which he may have to titrate against solution B. Half an hour later he arrives at a colour reaction which he has to demonstrate to his supervisor, and after two more (often blasphemous) hours, he achieves, if he is lucky, the production of a fine white crystalline powder, of which he then has to determine the solubility. It is this type of experiment, commonly stigmatized as 'cookery', which raises most of the questions regarding the value of practical work (Beard, 1970). It has its counterpart in other disciplines in which much emphasis is sometimes placed on the recording of nerve impulses, the collection of lymph, the sugar reactions of bacteria, and other similar matters, all of which might satisfactorily be dealt with by means of demonstrations. The argument in favour of such classes is that they teach the student the rudiments of experimental technique; without these he will be unable to understand the results obtained by other people, and to appreciate the difficulties inherent in their interpretation. The facts which are supplied to him to illustrate these principles may be forgotten, but the principles will remain. Once again we must conclude that these contentions are not proven; there have been no controlled investigations.

The proponents of the operational school of curricular reform point out very rightly that we should always be asking ourselves what the experiment is *for*, and attempting to define the primary aims of practical work. Is it to gain skill as an experimenter? Is it to see what difficulties are involved in practical work? Is it to rub home a point? The Hale Report (1964) suggests that the purposes served by a practical class may be summarized under five headings: to train students in manipulative skill; to introduce them to a range of techniques and instruments; to illustrate, supplement, and emphasize points from lectures or from private reading; to train students to write experimental reports, and to give them some sort of critical awareness of the nature and organization of a well-designed experiment.

In many places it has been decided that the main objective of practical classes ought to be to induce the student to think for himself—the appropriate slogan is, 'Make them use their own minds'—and to gain experience in the devising of experimental work and in the interpretation of the results. In order to achieve these objectives corporate experiments may be used. A problem is put to the class, which is then split up into groups to consider how it may best be attacked. Each group is then given a specific portion of the problem, and discusses it with an instructor. The members of the group formulate their own line of approach, which is approved by the instructor if it is feasible, and they then proceed to obtain the apparatus suitable for carrying it out. When they have achieved their results, these are put alongside the results obtained by other groups dealing with other portions of the problem, and a final discussion takes place at which the results are interpreted. Such a procedure undoubtedly must provide the student with an insight into the difficulties of experimentation, and give him the feeling that he is doing original work. But it has difficulties of its own. One of the most intractable of these is that the problem is broken down into such small parts that the student who is involved in only one of the component experiments has responsibility for only a minute fraction of the whole investigation, and his contribution may be swamped in the massive contribution of the remainder of the class. Accordingly, he may find it difficult to take an overall view of the whole affair, and in any case obtains very little personal experience except in the limited technique which his own group used. Even more serious is the immense amount of time and trouble which such experiments demand from the staff concerned. Even a simple problem has a habit of breaking down into an unwieldy number of components, and the organization of co-operative work is very difficult for all but the most experienced of staff. For this reason the technique has not spread very far beyond its originators.

Another fairly recent innovation is the provision of multipurpose laboratories, particularly in new medical schools. The basic reason for this is economy. As in the case of lecture theatres, it has been traditional for every department to have its own practical laboratory. In times of soaring building costs, such a practice is inherently wasteful, and becomes much more so when each laboratory is equipped with expensive instruments largely duplicating those found in other laboratories. The most obvious example is afforded by the microscopes which are often provided by several different departments. It is ludicrously bad housekeeping to store and service (say) 100 microscopes in each of the departments of biology, anatomy, pathology, and microbiology, together with many other microscopes in other departments less closely concerned with the study of microscopic structure. The obvious solution is to try to programme a single histological laboratory in such a way as to allow each department access to it, just as lecture theatres can be shared.

This feeling has been rationalized by some medical schools into an argument in favour of the educational value of such a device. It is claimed that the experience of doing practical work in several different departments makes the student fragment his experience into different 'subjects', so that he loses sight of the connexion between them. For example, the fact that the histology of a nerve trunk is examined in a building in one part of the campus, and its behaviour when stimulated is studied in another building elsewhere is said to make the student tend to separate them in his mind, instead of regarding them as two different aspects of the same thing. The conclusion is drawn that centralizing the practical work tends towards integration of knowledge [see p. 82], but here, as almost everywhere in education, medical or otherwise, there is no shadow of evidence.

What is more susceptible of proof is the difficulty of servicing and maintaining such equipment as microscopes in integrated multipurpose laboratories, and of apportioning blame when something goes wrong. Each department using such a laboratory is fully conscious that it alone looks after the microscopes properly and keeps them in good condition, and that any damage or working defect is thus attributable to one of the other departments. Bad feeling is at once widespread when one of the objectives is found to be broken, or when microscopes are left out on the bench, and the same sort of emotional problems arise that are common in universities where electron microscope facilities are shared among different departments. Where not only microscopical work, but chemical and functional experiments are done in the same laboratory, the difficulties are even greater. The bench heights required differ for different forms of activity, the housing of chemicals and instruments presents trouble, and the timetabling is extremely awkward, since one class must be cleared up before another can begin. For these and other reasons multipurpose laboratories are not a wholly satisfactory answer to the logistics of practical work, and few established medical schools are considering adopting them, though they are relatively common in new schools where building proceeds from scratch.

The important point in all preclinical practical work is to retain a firm sense of its purpose. 'Learning by doing' is an admirable slogan up to a point, but not all 'doing' involves learning, and there are many things that lectures, demonstrations, and films may do better than the student's own hands.

Clinical

If there are reservations about the value of practical work in the preclinical period, there are none about its value in the clinical period. Clinical skill is an essential attribute of any doctor who has to deal with patients, and the only discussion centres round how best to acquire it. Most medical schools have what they call 'an introductory clinical course' in which the principles of history-taking and of the examination of patients are taught to the entire class. Much of this introductory time is often entrusted to the department of psychiatry, in order that it can impart the basic importance of talking to the patient and eliciting accurately the story and symptoms of his illness. The physical examination of the patient is usually dealt with by clinical demonstrations, in which a long-suffering patient is examined in turn by individual students under the supervision of a physician or surgeon. This is tedious and repetitive work for a busy clinician, and the regrettable result is that such teaching is often done by the junior clinical staff, who may have little skill at exposition, and students are often left to pick up things as best as they can.

Nowadays, instruction in the matter of clinical signs and physical examination can often be helped enormously by the use of film or videotape. In this way the whole class can obtain the same indoctrination, and their subsequent progress is rendered much easier to plan. The phonocardiograph can play breath or heart sounds to the entire class, and does not get tired or testy, like even the most willing patient. Some schools have gone so far as to equip a lifelike mechanical dummy with various physical signs in order to avoid the undue handling of patients which otherwise inevitably occurs. By these and other approaches it is possible to give the student an adequate amount of preliminary information on what he should examine and how to examine it.[8] Inevitably, however, many matters cannot be demonstrated by such means. Practical work in the wards or in the sideroom beyond a certain stage becomes more a matter of apprenticeship than anything else, and the student learns by copying his seniors. As Samuel Butler said, 'An art can only be learned in the workshop of those who are winning their bread by it'.

In all cases where the care of patients and the teaching of students are mixed together, it is found that a few people are good at both, but most are good at one and not at the other. The appointment of a registrar, on whom much teaching of students, particularly at the elementary stage, may devolve, is usually decided without any reference to his possible capacity to' teach. This, of course, is only extending normal university practice into clinical medicine, but when so much

[8] In Leeds a computer has been called in to help students to learn clinical diagnosis (de Dombal, Hartley, and Sleeman, 1969; de Dombal, Horrocks, Staniland, and Gill, 1971). The machine is equipped with a number of files which provide a large variety of 'patients'; the responses of the computer guide the student to approach each 'case' in a logical and orderly fashion, progressively discovering more and more information. The system described is something of a cross between 'programmed learning' [see p. 126] and 'patient management problems' [see p. 153].

depends on people in this key position, it is unfortunate for the student if the registrar is more interested in research work or clinical care than he is in explaining things to junior students.

The taking of case notes is a practical operation which most medical schools insist that students shall perform in order to obtain practice in the difficult art of sorting out relevant and irrelevant factors. Case notes are therefore often called for, and the student may be assessed upon them. However, as with practice examination questions and preclinical essays, it is common to find that the case notes submitted are never returned with criticisms, so that the student never finds out where he has gone wrong. This is a basic mistake in teaching technique, and feedback on their practical work is essential if students are not to become discouraged.

The example afforded the student by his first clinical teachers is of the greatest importance. The transition from the 'scientific' part of the medical course to the 'humane' part is necessarily a difficult one, and cannot be made satisfactorily unless adequate patterns of behaviour are provided. The most generous and noble-minded exhortations in textbooks of psychiatry and social medicine pale into insignificance beside the observation of the application of these principles in everyday life. Even in these cynical and depressing days a student likes to have someone to look up to, someone whose behaviour he can respect, and from whom he can learn the principles of his future professional life. It is precisely in this respect that he is often disappointed. The pressure of work, the scientific advances, the administrative responsibilities—all these combine to make it easier for the clinician to be abrupt, mechanical, and uncommunicative when dealing with patients. In the film of James Hilton's book *Lost Horizon* the head of the lamasery in Tibet rephrased one of the world's most important principles in the two words, 'Be kind'. This is the main lesson that the student should learn in his clinical years, but it is only too evident that many students have difficulty in learning it, and the fault must be laid squarely on their teachers. Patients are often regarded as mere bundles of displaced electrolytes, and their personal problems and fears may be thought of as a tiresome accompaniment to a really interesting disease process.

The traditional formal ward round, in which patients are taught upon in the open ward, in the presence of teaching, nursing, and ancillary staff, together with a retinue of some 15 to 20 students,[9] is

[9] 'The worst lectures pale by comparison with the average teaching ward round, so often a display of bedside abracadabra to the tune of aching feet and wandering thoughts.' (Illingworth, 1968.)

on its way out, and the more humane practice of teaching in a side-room, with the consenting patient brought in for demonstration purposes, is taking its place (Hawkins, 1968). The old practice is not yet quite dead, however, and every now and then complaints against it are registered in the daily press. Hospital patients are on the whole extremely helpful and willing to advance the cause of medical education (Ogston and McAndrew, 1967), and a very great debt is owed to them by the medical profession (*Report of the Royal Commission*, 1968). Yet this good will is still sometimes eroded by unfair or heartless treatment on the part of a consultant, and there is no excuse whatever for this. It is intolerable, for example, that details of a poor prognosis should be discussed within the patient's hearing, or that he or she should be treated as a moron incapable of understanding the simplest information. The major complaint of patients in any teaching hospital today is that they receive inadequate information about their condition and about their future treatment. If a patient has the temerity during a ward round to ask the consultant for information, only too often he is put off with a non-committal remark, or outright rudeness. In this way the student learns that patients are not to be considered as human beings, and the inconsiderate or bad habits of the consultant are perpetuated in the next generation. The existence in Britain of a society for the protection of patients is a massive indictment of failure to communicate to students the elementary principles of regard for other people.

Every consultant should realize the imitative capacity of his juniors, and should take the necessary steps to inculcate, by his own behaviour, a sense of the importance of human factors, and to maintain the human sympathy which students naturally feel with those who are ill or distressed. Real compassion for the sick or troubled only comes in most cases after graduation, when the student has to handle such cases on his own.

The Royal Commission suggests the exploration of the relatively untried method of group clinical teaching. Instead of being attached to a given medical or surgical ward, the students are attached in small numbers to a group of teachers representing a spectrum of clinical and paraclinical skills. A group of this kind 'might include a surgeon, a physician, a pathologist, a radiologist . . . a general practitioner and a psychiatrist, and be supplemented as necessary by others . . .'. An arrangement of this kind, if practicable, could certainly contribute towards horizontal integration of clinical information, and give students an insight into the ways in which various forms of clinical practice interact with each other; the administrative difficulties are, at the moment, relatively unexplored.

But perhaps the most valuable form of practical work is still clinical clerking, in which a small group of students is attached to a particular ward or clinical unit and follows the patients admitted to this unit from the time of admission to the time of discharge. They are usually required to take the case-history, which is then criticized, and may assist in diagnostic procedures, write up case notes, witness any operations performed, and eventually visit the patients at home after discharge. Under ideal conditions all this may happen, but the reality is not always so praiseworthy. A great deal depends on the attitude towards students, not only of the senior medical staff, but of their juniors, and, perhaps above all, of the senior nursing staff. Clinical clerks are regarded by some sisters and staff nurses as a necessary evil, and are given little in the way of help or encouragement. Nevertheless, the clerking system, as the Royal Commission says, 'affords opportunities, especially in regard to the inculcation of attitudes, that cannot be so well provided in other ways'. The General Medical Council (1967) regards clinical clerkships as 'the indispensable method' of clinical teaching, and recommends that the student should be resident in the hospital or close to it for at least half the time spent in clerking.

Apprenticeship

The General Medical Council (1967) also recommends that the student should, in addition to his clerkship in hospital, spend a period of attachment to a general practitioner in order to obtain experience of types of illness which do not normally require hospital treatment. He sees how general practice is organized and learns about the services available to doctor and patient in the world outside the hospital.

This period is usually greatly appreciated by students; it gives them an insight into the branch of medicine which, for most of them, is the only branch of which they have had personal experience at the receiving end, and the contact with patients in their natural surroundings is stimulating and impressive. Here too, much depends on the practitioner to whom the attachment is made. Many of them go to immense trouble to make their students welcome and to help them in every way possible, and in such circumstances the experience is very valuable indeed.

THE PREREGISTRATION YEAR

The purpose of the preregistration year [see p. 8], which the General Medical Council (1967) now firmly includes under the heading of Basic Medical Education, is to extend the student's experience by providing an 'apprentice' year of supervised responsibility in hospital, without the necessity of working for examinations. In this year he acquires skill in practical procedures and is supposed to fit himself for the vocational training which follows registration. The Council considers that some such experience of responsibility should be given to students in their final university year, and sympathizes with medical schools which desire to free the final year from written examinations, as has already been done in Aberdeen. By this means 2 years of graduated supervised clinical experience can be provided instead of 1.

But the Council points out that there is almost universal disillusionment with the value of the preregistration year itself. Although some of the preregistration posts probably provide excellent supervised tuition and practical work, in too many 'the good habits of study and reflection which (it may be hoped) have already been formed can be irrecoverably dissipated in a year of unresting labour'. Not all preregistration posts are at present under the close supervision of the medical school in which the student has been educated, and in some of them the pressure of work is so great that medical education comes to an inevitable halt, though medical experience may pour in at an unassimilable rate. The present legal requirement is that the individual medical school should approve, on behalf of their graduates, the particular posts which they wish to fill, but the Council feels that this is not enough, particularly when some of these posts are a long way from the school, and suggests that some system of joint supervision among medical schools should be adopted so that education can be continued during the year. In this way graduates holding posts in a Hospital Region other than that associated with their own medical school would be supervised by the school of that Region.

The Council has made detailed recommendations about these posts. Six months should be spent in 'medicine' and 6 months in 'surgery' (midwifery may count as either surgery or medicine) but the time must be spent in posts affording *general* experience, in hospitals with adequate laboratory and other facilities, under the charge of consultants who are directly responsible for training. There should be at least one senior registrar in the department, or, if not, one or more registrars in residence. The graduate should not be responsible for more than 30 beds, and he should be allowed at least 6 hours weekly for educational purposes, apart from free time. Finally, there should be an educational programme including case conferences, seminars, and journal club meetings.

These proposals make heavy demands on the staffs of hospitals, which are not all geared to meet them. The 6 hours of educational time is often (so far) honoured in the breach, as are several of the other desiderata. As long as the National Health Service is chronically understaffed, so long will the preregistration year present an educational headache to those responsible for it, among whom must now be numbered the faculties of medicine whose products occupy its posts.

But worse is to come. With the expansion of student intake at present being forced on the medical schools [see p. 32], the number of graduates requiring placement in preregistration posts must rise. The number of suitable posts affording good educational experience is already very inadequate, and it is inescapable that others, still less suitable, will be pressed into service, or created to meet the demand. If proper training is to be afforded to graduates in this period of their basic medical education, a tremendous upheaval must occur in the attitude of the university medical schools towards the preregistration year, and extra facilities and teaching equipment, to say nothing of extra staff, will be needed.

STUDENT ADVICE AND GUIDANCE

Particularly in the early years of his course the student is often confused and worried by what appears to him to be a vast impersonal academic machine which operates without regard to his own difficulties and preoccupations. It is therefore very valuable for him to be able to obtain advice from a staff member who is directly concerned with his education, though preferably not with his academic assessment. To meet this need many universities now operate a 'regent' system, based on the concept of a 'moral tutor' at the ancient universities. All new students are allotted to a staff member who acts as a sort of ombudsman *cum* parent-substitute *cum* counsellor to those in trouble. Many of his flock may never consult him, but others may find the provision of such a helper very valuable indeed, particularly in the large classes which circumstances are thrusting upon the medical schools. From his regent the student may obtain advice on academic difficulties or personal problems; through him he may be put in touch with psychiatric help, and by him he may be enabled to discard some of his immature ideas and prejudices about university life, the practice of medicine, the value of work, and the division of the world into 'us' and 'them'.

In the clinical and preregistration period of basic medical education, advice on planning a career is particularly needed, and it is at this stage that the value of good relationships between clinicians and students or recent postgraduates is particularly apparent. Some schools have now undertaken the appointment of a postgraduate dean, whose office will function as a clearing house for information regarding careers and career posts, and such a system may well prove more efficient than the present dependence on haphazard personal contact.

7 Assessment

The greatest fool can ask more than
the wisest man can answer.

Colton

ASSESSMENT OF STUDENTS

Since the day when the first written paper was set, or the first oral
examination undertaken, people have been complaining about the
inequity, clumsiness, inadequacy, and inappropriateness of examinations in general. Yet they are still with us, and no better means has
yet been suggested of making the assessments which are almost
universally admitted to be necessary. The medical curriculum in
Britain inherited a heavy examination schedule as a legacy
from the days of the 'safe doctor', and even now this schedule
dominates the thinking of the students to the extent that passing
examinations is more important to them than learning how to be a
doctor.

The medical profession has been described as the most examination-
orientated in the world, and the blame for this has been attributed to
the students themselves, for they tend to take the view that a subject
cannot be important unless it is tested by examination.[1]

External

A university is in some ways similar to a manufacturer, for both turn
out branded products. Just as people rely on the quality of branded
articles, so they depend on the level of knowledge and competence
which the university certifies by the award of its degree. It follows
that universities have to test the quality of their products before
stamping them with their approval. In Britain the general public is as
yet in no position to form its own judgement on the value of such
tests, and it was largely for this reason that the General Medical

[1] L. G. Whitby, quoted in *Medical News Tribune*, 2 October 1970.

Council was set up [see p. 5], and charged with the duty of inquiring into the systems of assessment enforced by the different licensing bodies. The possession of a medical degree recognized by the Council guarantees a place on the Medical Register, and this is the criterion which is the safeguard of the public. The assessments employed by the various medical schools for the award of their degrees may differ qualitatively and quantitatively, but provided the Council is satisfied that they have investigated carefully the professional competence and skill of their graduates, this fact is immaterial. Other pathways to registration are provided by the external examinations set by the Conjoint Boards, either in London or in Scotland, and by the Society of Apothecaries. These examinations may be taken by students in any university, and it is possible for a student to fail his university degree examinations and still succeed in obtaining qualification for registration by passing the examinations set by one of these outside bodies. The numbers doing so are small, and the Royal Commission on Medical Education considers that all medical students should aim at the degree awarded by their own university.

The Royal Commission has also suggested that Britain should establish a Board, similar to the National Board of Medical Examiners [see p. 11] in America, which would supply standardized and tested examination questions to any medical schools that might wish to have an independent outside assessment of their students. Such an arrangement would allow comparisons to be drawn between standards of achievement in different medical schools, and would also provide an independent evaluation of any changes in performance following the introduction of educational experiments [see p. 172]. Discussions on ways and means have already been held, and specific proposals are now awaited.

Many students in British medical schools now sit the qualifying examinations set by the United States Educational Council for Foreign Medical Graduates at the time of their final examinations in their own school. Usually the examination is taken then because the student feels that he might wish to practise in America at some future date, and does not want to have to set about taking the examination later on. When Britain enters the European Economic Community all sorts of problems will undoubtedly present themselves regarding the external assessment of British graduates wishing to practise in Europe, and European doctors wishing to practise in Britain, and no doubt some universally applicable form of external examination will be worked out in the future [see p. 184].

Internal

The assessment procedures within a medical school not only provide a yardstick by which the General Medical Council can measure standards, they also determine the success or failure of the individual student. Exclusions based on failure must depend on adequate evidence, and the tests applied must be related to the suitability of the candidate to continue in a medical career. Exclusions must also occur as early as possible in the curriculum, because of the immense cost of allowing unsatisfactory students to continue. Regarded from this standpoint, the examinations and assessment procedures of the first 2 or 3 years have a much greater significance than those which are set in the later years, for by the end of the preclinical course the weaker students will theoretically have been weeded out, and the selected group which remains will be capable of dealing with the clinical work satisfactorily without having to be bothered with too great a load of assessment. The failure rates in the later stages of the curriculum are therefore much lower than they are in the earlier stages, and this is as it should be—not only for the crude reason of expense, but also because it is wholly desirable that someone who is not fitted for a career in medicine should be detected and excluded in time for him to take up an alternative career without having invested too much effort in the wrong direction.

In former days students were permitted to make repeated attempts to reach the required standard, but sheer economic necessity has forced most medical schools to allow them less latitude. A permissive view of student failure is, moreover, cumulative. The longer an unsatisfactory student is allowed to persist in his attempts to obtain a degree, the more difficult it becomes for the authorities to harden their hearts and expel him. So much so that a stage may be reached where a case could be made on purely compassionate grounds for him to carry on. If this case were to prevail, he might eventually obtain a totally undeserved degree, and find himself quite unable to compete in the hard and unsympathetic world outside the medical school. It therefore behoves the departments which encounter the student early in his career to be particularly careful about maintaining their standards of assessment strictly, and acting accordingly.

But here at once a difficulty presents itself. Most of the examinations set in the preclinical stage are necessarily concerned primarily with the work the candidate has been doing in the department or departments concerned; they are not, and cannot be, concerned with intangible factors such as the candidate's character, motivation, tact, kindliness, and ability to handle people. Yet these factors are of the greatest importance in determining the candidate's fitness to practise medicine. This problem has two diametrically opposed aspects. On the one hand, many are excluded on the grounds of academic weakness in subjects which play little part in the kind of medical career they would afterwards have chosen. The student with a vocation for psychiatry may fail in anatomy; the dedicated orthopaedic surgeon may be unable to cope with biochemistry. On the other hand, students who have an academic facility, but who are unsuited to clinical practice on the grounds of character defects, may be passed on to the clinical years, where, it is hoped, they can be dissuaded from embarking on a professional career in which their difficulties would prove a handicap to themselves and injurious to their patients; it is not always possible to ensure that this happens.

There is a considerable advantage in having a separate committee to decide on the disposal of a student who has failed an examination. The examiners merely report to this 'promotions' committee that the student has failed to come up to the expected academic standard, and the committee may then take into consideration the student's previous record and any mitigating circumstances such as illness, family troubles, or other problems. The student may be required to appear before the committee to explain the reasons for his failure, and the outcome can then be decided with much more knowledge of all the relevant facts than it is possible for the examiners to obtain. The membership of the committee may include representatives of several academic disciplines (usually including a psychologist or psychiatrist) as well as people with experience of student counselling.

However failures are dealt with, it is not surprising that clinicians should protest about the immense personal significance of the preclinical examinations, and that they should attempt to alter the system so that less depends on the results. It is widely believed that the worst ordeal a student has to face in his medical course is to be found in the examinations at the end of the preclinical period of the orthodox curriculum—examinations in anatomy, physiology, biochemistry, and sometimes pharmacology.[2]

The extreme solution to the problem is to abolish all forms of examination altogether and substitute a system of reports written by the departmental staffs on each student.[3] This solution, which is

[2] In 1970 a group of research workers seeking to elucidate physiological factors affecting the reaction to stress chose medical students undergoing their anatomy oral examination in order to investigate maximum strain (Bridges, 1970).
[3] For details of the methods employed, see Miller *et al.* (1961).

called continuous assessment (Heywood, 1969), is not in force in many schools, and suffers from a number of drawbacks. Only a small proportion of the students in a large class can become known to the teaching staff of a department with few teaching hours well enough for them to attempt to write any kind of meaningful report. If the difficulty is solved by making each staff member responsible for assessing the capabilities of a small group of students, those who fail may charge that the staff member concerned was partial or unfair in his report [see p. 110]. Again, junior staff, who usually have the opportunity to get to know the students best, may be reluctant to damn them by submitting a bad report. Students like to know how they are progressing,[4] and may actually enjoy being tested officially better than the fancied experience of being 'spied upon' by staff members who are going to write a report which will include deficiencies as well as proficiencies. In fact, some students may worry if they are not examined at intervals, for this system affords them the opportunity to make sure that they are on the right lines, and also gives them a short-term objective to work for.

Less drastic than complete abolition is the proposal that the terminal examinations, at the end of the course, should have a less portentous impact, and that more importance should be attached to performance in the intercurrent tests taken at intervals throughout the course. This solution, or something like it, is favoured both by the General Medical Council (1967) and by the Royal Commission on Medical Education, and is already in operation in many schools, both in Britain and elsewhere: it is usually called intercurrent or intermittent assessment. In some places it has been taken so far that terminal assessment has been dispensed with, and students are now passed or failed on the basis of their intercurrent performance (Trethowan, 1970). It is true that a single terminal examination, lasting perhaps 3 hours, affords such a small sample of the total material dealt with during the course that an element of luck enters into the result. On the other hand, it is considerably easier to pass a series of small examinations, each relating to a particular segment of the course, than it is to accumulate and retain enough knowledge and skill to pass an examination on the whole content of the subject at one given time. To those who complain about the strain on the student involved, it may be said that a doctor in clinical practice never knows what problems his next patient is going to present; he cannot afford to say to a sufferer from acute appendicitis or a

[4] Even in childhood the desire to find out how you are getting on is very strong; 7-year olds like being examined and ask, 'Did I get 100?' (Gesell and Ilg, 1949).

ruptured spleen, 'I am afraid you have a condition which I have not studied in the last 2 months; I must ask you to wait while I look it up'. Sooner or later the doctor must learn to keep considerable masses of information in his head, and this can probably best be done by insisting that he learns how to do this from an early stage in his training. Those places in which the intercurrent assessment results are used as a substitute for the terminal assessment run the risk of lowering the standards on which they make decisions.

Some medical schools give a fixed percentage of the total marks to the intercurrent assessment, and the remainder to a terminal examination. If the percentage allotted to the intercurrent assessment is high, it is possible to achieve the pass marks without getting any marks at all in the final examination. In one such case a student whom I examined in topographical anatomy knew absolutely nothing when confronted with a living body at her final oral, for which she obtained nought. Yet she passed. Another objection is that students who know that by piling up marks during the year the final examination can be made to lose its terrors may develop an unhealthy interest in marks as an end in themselves rather than as a shorthand method of saying 'good', 'indifferent', or 'bad'.

Another difficulty is that of interpreting the marks awarded during intercurrent assessment. The same average mark can be obtained by very different kinds of people, as TABLE 1 indicates, and some of these are more deserving of promotion than others. For example,

TABLE 1

PATTERNS OF INTERCURRENT ASSESSMENT
(PASS MARK 50 PER CENT)

STUDENT	1	2	TEST 3	4	5	6	AVERAGE	STUDENT COMMENT	STAFF DIAGNOSIS
A	50	50	50	50	50	50	50	None	Plodder
B	20	30	50	60	70	70	50	None	Initial confusion
C	60	50	55	10	60	65	50	Rugby club dinner	Rugby club dinner
D	30	40	30	40	80	80	50	Suddenly came to me	Painful interview with Professor
E	60	60	60	30	30	60	50	Couldn't concentrate	Row with girl friend
F	40	30	40	40	30	30	35	I know it, but . . .	Lacks ability and insight
G	60	50	40	30	20	10	35	None	Real trouble
H	15	Abs	10	Abs	Abs	5	5	Dedicated to medicine	Not interested

many people confronted by a new subject are at first confused and bewildered, and initially do badly; only later do they get a grasp of the situation, and their marks may show a steadily rising curve. Others, who are not interested, or who discover outside attractions, may show a curve which is exactly the reverse of this. A complicated weighting system may thus be needed, which makes the whole thing far too rigid and inelastic.

For these reasons it seems preferable to attach a qualitative rather than a quantitative value to the intercurrent assessments, and to make the final examination count for rather more than performance during the year. In general, there are two groups of satisfactory students; those who work steadily throughout the year, and those who do relatively less during the course, but are able to revise the material satisfactorily in a short high-pressure burst just before the terminal examination. It seems desirable that both types should be given the advantage which their particular method of working allows them.[5] For this reason intercurrent assessments, which might penalize the latter group if they were used both for and against students, are used by some schools in their favour but not against them. In this way the student who leaves it until the last few weeks to do the work is not penalized, provided that he can baffle the examiners on the great day.

The value of intercurrent assessment is that it allows discussion of the results with the teachers, who also have a feedback on what parts of the course have failed to penetrate to the students' understanding. A department which has no intercurrent examinations is thus at a disadvantage compared with those which do, but it is important to add the proviso that discussion of the results becomes difficult or impossible if multiple choice questions are used, and this is one of the disadvantages of this form of examination [see p. 150].

Whatever method of assessment is used, it cannot be too strongly urged that its rationale and details must be clearly and unequivocally made known to the students when they embark on the course. This point was forcibly put in a paper prepared by the National Union of Students in 1968, and though their criticism was not specifically directed towards the medical faculty, it is undoubtedly true that students are all too often mystified by the systems adopted by different departments. If they have just left a department in which essays, projects, notebooks, and performance in seminars count for nothing in the final assessment, they may well be surprised and justifiably

---

[5] One might like to believe that those who work steadily will retain the information longer, but there is no evidence for this supposition.

aggrieved when they find out (too late) that all these points are used, perhaps with a heavy weighting, by the teachers under whose care they now find themselves, and who have not bothered to notify them of the different system.

No other topic, with the possible exception of childbirth, is so liable to surround itself with gossip, superstition, and pure unadulterated fancy, as the behaviour of examiners (Sinclair, 1955), and if students are not given concrete information about assessment they will at once set about constructing a framework of delusions which will enable them to hold the unknown at bay. Indeed, any information must be written down rather than read out, and must be worded with legal precision; if not, word of mouth will have distorted the procedure within a week so that it becomes wholly unrecognizable.

It is also very desirable that the standards required of the student should be the same throughout the course. A student who passes an intercurrent examination should know that, provided he keeps up a similar standard, he should pass at the final examination also.

It is often urged that a student's knowledge should not be tested at a time when his mind is affected by the crisis of a major examination. In medicine this argument has less to commend it than in other faculties. It is one of the features of medical practice that it presents a continuing series of minor (or even major) crises, and if a student is so disturbed by the thought of an examination that he is unable to perform properly in it, it is surely likely that he will be unable to cope satisfactorily with the stresses and strains he will encounter after qualification (Henn, 1951).

So much attention has recently been devoted to the iniquities and inequities of the examination system in the medical curriculum, and so much effort spent in attempting to reduce the examination load that we are in danger of forgetting that the failure rate over the whole course in medicine is only two-thirds of the average for university undergraduates (*British Medical Journal*, 1968). Only two students in every 23 fall by the wayside, and, considering the difficulties of student selection (Sinclair, 1955, 1956a) this figure does seem to indicate that the horrors of the examination system are perhaps not quite so overpowering as they have been represented. After all, one has only to look round the medical profession to see that quite ordinary people have survived them. It is also interesting that the 'second professional examination' in anatomy, physiology, and biochemistry, which was the target for so much vituperation on the part of medically qualified critics of the orthodox curriculum, escaped from criticism almost unscathed in the *Report on*

Undergraduate Medical Education made by the British Medical Students' Association in 1957.

Examination Format. Where so much depends on the examination system, the form taken by the examinations is of paramount importance. Many forms of experimental examinations are practised in different medical schools—objective examinations of various kinds, written papers in which the questions are given out ahead of time, 'open-book' papers, simulated clinical examinations [see p. 153]. But throughout the country the main emphasis falls on orthodox essay-type written papers, multiple choice objective examinations, practical (particularly clinical) assessment, and oral examinations. Both the essay question and the multiple choice question have their advantages and drawbacks (Marshall, 1953; Sinclair, 1953, 1955; Miller *et al.*, 1961), but at present the latter is steadily gaining ground in Britain, partly because some people feel that the use of essay questions tends to penalize those who cannot express themselves easily and fluently in English,[6] but mainly because of the increase in student numbers. When an examiner has 150 papers to mark, each consisting of five essay questions, he tends to think kindly of a method in which the whole of the marking and percentaging of the results can be done by a machine.

It is well known that essay questions are unreliable, and that different examiners will give them different marks, that they sample a small area of the total territory which could be presented, and that they are tedious and time-consuming to mark (Hubbard and Clemans, 1961; Beard, 1970). But in view of the present apparently uncritical acceptance of multiple choice questions, it is as well to look briefly at the drawbacks which an exclusive reliance on this form of examination entails (Marshall, 1953, 1956*a*, 1958*a*; Walton and Drewery, 1967; Gibson, 1969). In the first place, at no time is the student given the opportunity of writing down his views on any subject at some length. He is never encouraged to assemble his knowledge into coherent form, nor is he able to stray outside the confines of the question in front of him. The better the student, the more difficult he finds it to answer multiple choice questions satisfactorily to himself, since if the distractors are of any value, they must have some semblance of plausibility. The more a student knows about a given topic, the less

[6] As Churchill is reported to have said, writing to an admiral whose dispatches were not written to his satisfaction, 'Mere jottings of passing impressions hurriedly put together without sequence, and very often with marked confusion, are calculated to give an impression the reverse of that which is desirable.'

definite and clear cut become the answers, so that he wishes to qualify every statement he is asked to assent to with provisos and exceptions. This he is not allowed to do. On the other hand, a student who may know little about the subject, but who has been brought up from childhood on multiple choice questions, may be able to perform very satisfactorily and pass the examination, although his knowledge is much inferior. I well remember visiting a distinguished American anatomist at the time when the National Board papers in anatomy[7] were being sat in his department. He and his staff answered the questions out of interest, and it emerged afterwards that they would all have done badly, even though the students whom they had taught did very well.

There are difficulties over making allowance for the effects of guessing (Husak, 1968; Harden, Lever, and Wilson, 1969), and mechanical difficulties over the machine-reading of the marks made by inexperienced students (Lennox, 1967).[8] Another objection to the objective format is that the student's performance cannot be discussed with the teacher afterwards, nor can the reasons for his failure be given. All that can be said is that he did not know a satisfactory amount about this or that aspect of the subject. But perhaps the most serious criticism of the multiple choice examination as used in Britain at the moment is that the majority of the questions are the productions of amateurs. Everyone fancies himself as a composer of objective questions, and some of those recently included in postgraduate examinations reveal considerable ignorance about the whole process of setting, combining, and evaluating such questions. When properly compiled, as by the National Boards organization in America, an objective paper can be a searching trial of the student's factual knowledge, and can also explore his understanding and some of his deductive reasoning powers. But when the questions are set without a full knowledge of the procedure required, and marked without a knowledge of the statistical difficulties involved, they are often of very little use (Miller *et al.*, 1961; Sanderson, 1969).

Nevertheless, multiple choice and true/false examinations have several great advantages. They can be machine-marked and analysed

[7] The National Boards examinations in the United States have had the multiple choice format for nearly 20 years (Stokes, 1967), and an independent organization (Pre Test Service Inc.) is now offering a practice examination comprised of a series of test questions similar to those of the National Boards. The student taking part in them receives a confidential score showing how his performance relates to the other students taking the Pre Test examination.

[8] Towers (1969) has recently pointed out that marking machines do not care for answer sheets with chewing gum on them; this must be counted a defect of the system.

by computer (Diament and Goldsmith, 1970; Lennox and Lever, 1970). They can be stored in a question bank (Buckley-Sharp and Harris, 1970), and indeed several American institutions, such as the State University of Iowa, have had examination centres for the last 20 years; each department requiring an examination merely contacts the centre and a multiple choice examination in its discipline is produced. The results, unlike those from essay questions, can be statistically compared without serious objection, providing the marking technique is identical in each case. Hence the growing use of such examinations for comparing student performance under different circumstances. One of the dangers in this lies in the fact that by the time the results have been reduced to means and standard deviations flashed out by an electronic calculator we have got quite a long way from what the students were actually asked, how they were asked it, the possible misunderstandings inherent in the process, and the possible errors in the method of marking. 'Objective' examinations are in fact not objective at all, for their setting and interpretation are very subjective indeed (Marshall, 1956a), and the fact that the marks can be manipulated by the statistician should not blind us to this fact.

Oral examinations are very commonly used in the faculty of medicine, and frequently serve to provide the casting vote for success or failure. Yet they are just as subject to error as any essay paper (Eysenck, 1953; McGuire, 1966; Colton and Peterson, 1967; Wilson et al., 1969), and those who are confident of their ability to sort people out by an interview technique of this kind suffer from a groundless optimism. Nevertheless, oral interviews are an essential part of every clinical test, and indeed of the working life of every clinician. It is very desirable, therefore, to see how the student performs in conversation, even if the assessment made is highly subjective, so long as too much weight is not placed upon the result relative to the candidate's other performances.

Although practical examinations are not so often required of the student in the preclinical phase of the curriculum as they used to be 50 years ago, clinical examinations are still strongly practical in nature. In the days when every newly qualified graduate was supposed to be a 'safe doctor', the final examination was intended to be a test of the candidate's capacity to handle various types of clinical situation. After writing essay papers in three or four major subjects, the student was confronted with a selection of patients, often specially imported into the wards for the occasion, and required to exhibit his clinical skill by examining, diagnosing, and prescribing for them. In most places the format of the final examination has altered very little since then, but there seems to be good reason why it should now be modified. It is surely absurd that in an era when integration is the watchword, students should still be examined in several disintegrated subjects, and that they should be asked to report on such monstrosities as 'long surgical cases' and 'short medical cases', instead of just on sick people. It is as though the patient in bed had a label tied to his big toe stating, 'I am a medical case, and my condition can only be discussed with a physician', or 'I am a surgical outpatient, and you must use only your surgical knowledge in dealing with me'. The student acts according to the format of the examination. Thus, if he is to take his 'surgery clinical' he goes prepared with his notes on surgery and surgical pathology, as well as with his knowledge of the foibles and preferences of the internal examiner and what he has heard of the prejudices of the external. On the following day, when he is confronted by an examination in clinical medicine or in paediatrics, he alters his tactics to suit the new situation. But patients in practice do not have such little labels tied on their big toes, and the student must be prepared to bring to the fore at one and the same time his knowledge of surgery, medicine, anatomy, biochemistry, pharmacology, and so on, in order to deal satisfactorily with the total clinical situation presented by the individual patient. To separate out the various facets of clinical management of patients is thus an unsatisfactory preparation for clinical practice in the wards or outside the hospital.

There is an intangible entity known as clinical competence, which can be applied equally well to surgical, medical, or other types of 'case'. It is therefore not unreasonable that the student should be asked to examine a patient—category unspecified—in his clinical finals, and that he should not know beforehand whether he will be subjected to questioning by a physician, a surgeon, or a specialist in some branch of clinical work. The capacity to handle a clinical situation, which such an examination can assess, can be separated from the specific knowledge of the various 'subject' components of the final years of the curriculum, which may be tested satisfactorily in short answer examination questions or in orals given by the specialist concerned.

In clinical examinations each candidate may have a different patient to examine. There is thus little uniformity, and it is difficult to ensure fairness. Some lucky students may be faced with a perfectly clear cut condition like a recurrent dislocation of the shoulder, while others may be confronted with a chronic pancreatitis in which the symptoms and signs are difficult to elicit and interpret. Again, some patients are very forthcoming, and through much practice, will confide their entire history in ringing phrases of crystal clarity, while others adopt the attitude of not giving anything away because that is what the student is supposed to be finding out; a third group either cannot or will not say anything at all. It is for such reasons that attempts have recently been made to simulate a clinical examination. The most effective of these simulations, which have been called patient management problems (McGuire, 1963, 1965; McCarthy and Gonnella, 1967), emanate from Professor George Miller's department in the University of Illinois. Each student is presented with a printed booklet containing a preliminary description of a clinical situation. The text then asks how he wishes to proceed, and according to the choice he makes, he is directed to an answer booklet in which further information about the case is masked by a layer of opaque material. He scrapes off this overlay in the places corresponding to his way of handling the situation, and finds clinical data such as the blood pressure, blood chemistry, pupil reactions, etc. Further instructions then lead him to scrape off more material elsewhere, and so to discover progressively more and more data. If he asks for a radiograph or an electrocardiogram a miniature print is provided. Having made a diagnosis he will be directed to follow a similar procedure in regard to treatment and perhaps to prognosis. If he makes a serious mistake in handling the case, the 'patient' may 'die' on his hands.

While these problems simulate a clinical situation, sometimes extremely well, and engage the candidate's emotions as well as his intellect (Williamson, 1965), the chief difficulty in using them in Britain lies in their expense. They are useful for specific investigations [see p. 160], but have a more restricted general applicability. Nevertheless, patient management problems test more than factual recall, more than mere understanding of the subject, and in the future it seems possible that an extension of this method may yet be devised to test attitudes as well.

It is at present quite impracticable to urge that the examination system should be abandoned, and the alternative is surely to investigate more closely the form of the examinations which are used. So long as students prepare for the examination and not for the medical profession, so long will the form and content of the examinations exert an incalculable effect on medical education. If students work for examinations, altering the examinations can alter the way they work, and this provides an educational weapon the force of which is as yet scarcely explored. If the examination set is one which tests factual recall, then the students will set to work remembering facts.

If the examination demands understanding, students will find it necessary to develop this quality, or face rejection. If each department (and indeed the whole faculty) only knew with precision what it wanted, and adjusted the examinations accordingly, it might give a new and broader meaning to the old saying that the main purpose of an examination has been fulfilled when the students sit down at their examination desks (Charvat, McGuire, and Parsons, 1968).

As a beginning, we ought to insist that every examiner defines in detail his objectives in framing the questions he asks. Written or objective questions may be composed so as to measure knowledge, comprehension, application, analysis, synthesis, and evaluation (Cowles, 1954; Miller, 1962). Yet, as Miller concludes, 'Only rarely do certifying examinations in medical school go beyond the second of these six levels, and this is true whether the essay or objective examination form is used'.

The examiner must ask himself exactly what skills, attributes, and information the particular examination under scrutiny *ought* to test (Bull, 1956; Miller *et al.*, 1961; Charvat, McGuire, and Parsons, 1968; Dudley, 1969). This operational view of assessment is only too often completely lacking, and questions are set unthinkingly because they 'make a good question' (Sinclair, 1955), because they are easy to mark, or simply because they have been used elsewhere and look interesting.[9]

Having established his objectives, and only then, the examiner should consider what format of examination will best fit them. If it is factual recall he is after, multiple choice questions may be adequate; if, as is usual, he is looking for more than this—say, the ability to argue a point or to set down a reasonable discussion of controversial material—he will have to employ other methods in addition, perhaps an oral confrontation or an essay paper. If these methods are used, they should be used for the particular purpose intended, and not

---

[9] An admirable statement of general examination objectives was made by an anonymous 'medical student' in a pamphlet directed to the Edinburgh professors and published in 1890: '. . . the examiners ought to keep steadily in view, in the questions they ask, simply and solely the candidate's capacity to practise his profession in a reasonably intelligent manner, worthy of the University. Let them insist, not on proficiency in a showy, but practically worthless appearance of knowledge, whether theoretical or practical; but on a certain moderate standard of *intelligent* acquaintance with the subject *in its main outlines*, and in a clear consciousness of ignorance where ignorance exists, as it must with regard to countless matters which a medical student has not the time to study, or which have not yet been successfully investigated. And let them not shirk, as they almost everywhere do at present, their full responsibility, but reject without exception all those whom they believe not to have a sufficient *grasp* of their work.'

merely to duplicate information already satisfactorily covered.[10]
Charvat, McGuire, and Parsons (1968) present the advantages and
drawbacks of each type of examination, and list critical performance
requirements for physicians, giving some indication of how they
might be tested; Heywood (1969) has provided a useful chart
indicating some of the factors influencing the assessment of academic
ability by various means.

It is at least encouraging that much more interest is nowadays
being shown in the methods of assessment available to university
teachers, and that a substantial research literature is at last beginning
to develop (Cox, 1967; Beard, 1969). Miller (1962) wonders whether
'our preoccupation with teaching may not have obscured the more
pressing issue of learning. If we have confidence in the devices we
employ to measure competence in the several areas of our interest,
need we be very concerned about how this competence was achieved,
whether in 3 years or 4, in 200 hours or half that many, in our classrooms and laboratories or in the student's own library and study? If
we do not have confidence in these tools of measurement would it
not be more profitable to devote more of our energies and resources
to their improvement before further shaking up the course of study
or establishing new time limits for exposure to instruction, the outcome of which will always be uncertain if our appraisals are
imprecise?'

External Examiners. The principle that students should be examined,
not only by those who had a hand in teaching them, but also by a
visiting examiner from another educational institution, has been
firmly established in Britain for many years, though in America it
does not appear to be thought necessary. It is, naturally, expensive,
for the external examiner has to be paid his fee for examining, and
must be transported free of charge from one place to another; this
must be done in reasonable comfort, or he will not be very keen to
repeat the experience. Yet the advantages so outweigh the expense
that external examiners are flown in multitudes over great distances
every year to examine in strange places, while their own departments
in turn receive visitors of the same kind.

Examining is a difficult job, and two heads are better than one.
Indeed, the General Medical Council (1967) stipulates that 'at least

---

[10] McGuire (1966), who investigated oral examinations held by a Speciality Board,
found that most questions related to factual knowledge, 'although there is virtually
universal agreement that factual knowledge is best evaluated with a written objective
examination'.

two assessors' should take part in all examinations. But if the two heads are both local ones, and if the student is examined only by those who taught him, he may come to believe that personal factors may sway the examiner's judgement, and he is therefore anxious not to create a bad impression by drawing attention to himself during the course. He is careful not to ask questions about his difficulties, for this may expose his ignorance, and he may even exert himself to keep out of the way of the departmental staff as much as possible.[11] He may come to look on his teachers as potential enemies rather than potential friends, and studies their opinions and quirks with care so that he will say only what he thinks will propitiate them.

At the same time the head of the department may be unwilling to mete out praise or blame as he feels he ought, because he fears he may be thought prejudiced. He may find himself in an awkward position when called upon to pronounce an unfavourable judgement upon the son or daughter of one of his personal friends or acquaintances. Finally, he may not like having to set all the questions in the examination, because he thinks that the students may then feel obliged to regurgitate uncritically only those opinions which they believe him to hold.

These problems can all be satisfactorily solved by sharing the burden of examining the class with a man who has had no contact with the students beforehand, and will have none afterwards. The student's work is then assessed by two inquisitors, one who is completely impartial but lacks knowledge of his work during the year, and another who knows his personal difficulties more intimately, and can bring his knowledge to bear in case of difficulty. Such a situation comes as near as appears practicable to the ideal of tempering justice with mercy.

An interchange of examiners does much to ensure a common standard of professional training throughout the Commonwealth, and encourages mutual confidence in the competence of professional men produced by different universities. The use of external examiners is even more important where very substantial modifications have been made in the orthodox curriculum. In a situation like this it is more than possible that the staff may be blinded with enthusiasm for new teaching methods or innovations, and that they could fail to see some of the deficiences which these might produce in the professional

---

[11] Miller *et al*. (1961) refer to the 'passion for anonymity' which characterizes the American medical student: 'A passion born of the belief that his progress towards the goal of graduation is less likely to be blocked if he remains essentially unidentified for four years.'

education of the students who are being experimented on. The test of success or failure of such modifications comes at the end of each year, when the students face their annual examinations, and it is most desirable to find out how they stand up to comparison with the students in more orthodox schools elsewhere. Most external examiners are also in a position to comment on what is going on in several other medical schools which they have recently visited. In this way the success or failure of new methods can become widely disseminated among the medical schools which have embarked on curricular reorganization.

Grades and Compensations. At the end of each academic year the examiners' committee meets to decide who has passed safely through the academic year and who must be referred to the promotions committee [see p. 144] for a decision as to their disposal. The information available from each department to the examiners' committee usually consists of a single letter grade ranging from 'A' (excellent) to 'F' (outright failure), often supplemented by a student 'profile' which gives in detail his performance in any essays, quizzes, tutorial classes, etc. These may or may not contribute to the grade, the major components in which are performance in the final battery of examinations and performance in intercurrent written, oral, or practical examinations throughout the year.

Usually, grading systems include provision for compensation—that is, an arrangement whereby a creditable performance in one 'subject' can allow a borderline failure in another subject to be converted into a pass. Such a system immediately introduces arguments about the weight to be placed on a grade from a particular department. For example, a student who has a borderline failure in a subject which only occupied 10 teaching hours during the year will readily be compensated if he has done well in two major subjects. But a failure in one of the major subjects is often felt to require more solid reasons for compensation than a reasonable pass in the minor subject. Again, complicated rules have to be introduced about multiple compensations. If four subjects are involved, can an 'A' in one of them compensate for two borderline failures among the others?

And so on: all sorts of 'regulations for the guidance of examiners' very rapidly multiply to cover over the fact that the examiners are dealing with a set of subjectively derived letters of the alphabet, depending on differently interpreted standards, and that they are required to sum these up into another all-embracing subjective judgement. Examiners are only human, though students often think otherwise, and they are faced with an unpleasant duty in having to weigh university standards and the welfare of the public (both rather abstract concepts at such a time) against the distress and disappointment—often even hardship—of the rejected candidate, who is a very personal presence, and may be well known and well liked by everybody concerned. Yet these decisions must be made, and though injustices are inevitable, the presence of external examiners [see p. 155] helps to reduce them to a minimum.

A strong body of opinion, led by Marshall (1953, 1954, 1958*b*, 1968), believes that any form of grading is unnecessary and may actually be harmful (Sinclair, 1955; Goldstein, 1958). This is certainly so when the grade symbol is made paramount instead of being looked on merely as a shorthand expression of opinion. Basically, all that is necessary is to be able to say, 'This student was satisfactory; that one was not', and to be able to support this with reasons. But if the assessment is to be used for compensation, or as part of an integrated examination result, or for the purpose of awarding a prize or a scholarship, then this bald statement is not enough. *How* satisfactory (or unsatisfactory) was the student? What weight shall we place on the result? The only way out of making quantitative judgements of this kind is to abolish compensation, prizes and scholarships, and the first of these, at least, is not often done in Britain nowadays.[12]

But at least the errors inherent in using percentage marks as though they were mathematically derived instead of being mere shorthand notations (Sinclair, 1955) is now being widely realized, and absurdities such as giving a candidate a mark of $43\frac{1}{2}$ per cent are no longer common. Whatever system is used, it is presumptuous to think in much more detailed terms than 'excellent', 'creditable', 'pass', 'borderline', and 'fail'. These can be given letters or figures for convenience's sake, but further subdivision is undesirable.

It must be added that for the great majority of passes and for most of the failures the verdict is unanimous: it is only a small number of failures who generate difficulties, and a great deal of time may be devoted to detailed consideration of these cases.

Marshall (1953, 1954, 1958*b*, 1968) has always maintained that grading can be avoided if teachers are willing to spend a very little extra time in writing down a brief summary of their opinions about every student. Even a single word may convey much more than the

---

[12] Bender (1969) found that, in the United States, grading on a letter or numerical system caused more emphasis to be placed on grades as an end in themselves than a simple pass/fail system. Both students and staff preferred the latter procedure, yet about half the schools studied operated a letter/numerical system.

bald letter of the alphabet for which it substitutes. Naturally no opinion is worth anything at all unless the author of it is known, and these 'profiles' are always signed. A similar system has been tried for some time at Pittsburgh (Cowles, 1965) and elsewhere (Geertsma and Chapman, 1967) in the clinical years of the medical course, and something like it seems to be envisaged by the Royal Commission (1968). The difficulties of such a procedure have already been stressed [see p. 145].

ASSESSMENT OF STAFF

In the Alice in Wonderland atmosphere surrounding present-day tertiary education it has been proposed that teaching skill shall be rewarded by extra payment. We are all aware that some people are good at teaching and that others are bad, but to attempt to quantify abstract qualities on a financial scale which compares the performance of a teacher teaching one subject with that of another teaching a different one is to attempt an impossibility. Some Vice-Chancellors have sensibly decided to let the idea alone, but others have entered upon this sisyphean labour by means of student questionnaires.

In some American medical schools students are regularly asked their opinions of the individual members of the teaching staff; their personalities, helpfulness, approachability, good temper, and general skill at putting difficult points across are all listed on scales ranging from excellent to atrocious. This exercise may occasionally be of some help to the staff members, who are thereby enabled to correct some of their worst technical faults. But to ask students to assess staff members for the purpose of awarding them extra payment is to reduce the concept to the lowest common denominator (Marshall, 1969b; Beard, 1970). The teacher many British students like best is the one who dictates notes slowly, so that every word can be written down, who tells them exactly what is important and what is not, who explains every difficulty in detail as he comes to it, who does not stray outside the strict confines of his 'subject', and who sets perfectly straightforward examination questions spelled out in words of one syllable and demanding only a knowledge of facts. Students do not like being made to think on their own, or to read round the subject; they like being spoon-fed, as they have been at school for so many years. In short, popular teaching is seldom the same as good teaching, though occasionally the two may coexist in a specially gifted individual.

The day that psychology develops to the point where students can infallibly assess intangible attributes of character and personality and assign numerical values to them will be the day it is proper to begin thinking of differential pay for relative teaching capacity.

ASSESSMENT OF CURRICULA

For 20 years there has been talk in Britain about establishing new curricula, and for 12 it has been possible to do so. In this last period many new curricula have been evolved, and some have been put into action. The changes proposed have often been quite radical and far-reaching, and have been made in order to counteract some supposed defect in the qualities and performance of the graduates of the particular school concerned. It may well be that drastic changes in quality and performance have been effected, but we shall never know, for not the slightest attempt has been made to evaluate the results of the changes made. The only British school that has made a beginning in this direction is Aberdeen, where patient management problems and multiple choice questions have been used to demonstrate that it is possible to evaluate the results of changing the curriculum, even though on a fairly elementary level (Sinclair, 1972). This particular experiment was faulty in that not every student took part, but it is to be hoped that other schools may follow suit and provide us with our first real information about what happens when a British educational pattern is changed.[13]

It is quite extraordinary that in a faculty whose members are trained to evaluate evidence and to insist on full controls for every experimental modification of diet or treatment, gigantic schemes of reorganization, which may affect the future lives of hundreds of doctors and their patients, should be embarked upon without even the smallest attempt to find out whether the results are good or bad. Admittedly, only an imperfect evaluation is possible in the present state of our knowledge (Sinclair, 1955; Jacobson, 1967), but factual knowledge can be adequately investigated (Levit, 1967), and patient management problems afford a means of evaluating something which comes very near to clinical skill. At least they are better than complete ignorance, with which most schools appear to be satisfied.

Another method of investigating curricula is the postgraduate survey; the products of a given medical school are circulated at a given

13 The school at Hamilton, Ontario, has indicated its intention to try (Campbell, 1970).

time after qualification, and asked their opinion of the medical course they underwent in relation to the occupation they subsequently took up. Two of the most comprehensive of recent investigations of this kind are those of Mair (1955) and McAndrew, Dawson, and Ogston (1970) dealing with Aberdeen graduates. While a survey can give a general impression, it suffers from several inherent defects. In the first place, the opinions relate to the state of the curriculum several years ago, when what is wanted is information on its *present* defects and advantages. Secondly, so diverse are the needs and occupations of the graduates that, as a rule, no firm conclusions can be arrived at; their memories of what they actually went through are often faulty, or coloured by subsequent experience, and may often be prejudiced in favour of or against a particular subject for reasons quite apart from its content.

While the major changes wrought by alteration of the curriculum remain uninvestigated, minor points are often studied by question- naire.[14] Thus, the students passing through an altered preclinical course may be circulated with a sheet asking them for comments and suggestions for modification. Committees are formed to discuss the results of specific changes, perhaps the substitution of tutorials for lectures; the faculty may debate such matters as the unfortunate effects of altering the pattern of teaching on the working hours of staff. But all these matters are decided pragmatically, on insufficient evidence, and according to the prejudices of those most nearly involved. In my view, the immense amount of work involved in establishing a new curriculum in substitution for an old one can only be justified if a specific research programme designed to evaluate the proposed changes is established well ahead of their implementation, so as to allow time for an adequate control investigation before the upheaval begins.

[14] The fact that formulating a questionnaire is a job for an expert is too often over- looked.

8 Introducing a New Curriculum

Every public action which is not
customary either is wrong, or, if it is
right, is a dangerous precedent. It
follows that nothing should ever be
done for the first time.

Francis Cornford

DISCUSSION AND DECISIONS

The first step towards introducing a new curriculum is the appointment of a planning committee. In an established school the composition of this committee is a matter for considerable debate and
anxiety. The members are usually drawn from among the more
senior members of the faculty, whose seniority may have been
achieved, through the passage of time, in several different ways, not
all of which involve much teaching. Some are good committee men
or useful administrators, others have a wide range of experience, and
others are eminent in their chosen branch of the profession. It thus
quite often happens that the committee may contain many people
whose experience of day-to-day teaching of undergraduates is out-of-
date. Moreover, those who are still engaged in it may, by the very
virtue of their distinction in their own field, have little knowledge of
current developments in other fields [see p. 71]. The members are
also, by definition, men who were keen enough academically to pursue their studies to the point where they were given a senior teaching
appointment; the schemes they formulate may for this reason have a
tendency to assume that all students are of a similar stamp, and to
take less than due account of the behaviour of the less than average
student.

The school will contain people who are anxious for 'progress' at
any price, and also people who are intensely conservative. In between
there is a body of floating voters who may be swayed one way or the
other. It is usually the reformers who press for the institution of the

committee, and as a result they find themselves members. The faculty will probably wish to counterbalance the excesses which they suspect these members of harbouring, and are therefore likely to appoint one or more traditionalists to act as a brake on some of the wilder ideas; in this it will be following the maxim laid down by Cornford (1908) that in academic affairs nobody should ever be allowed to act 'without first consulting at least 20 other people who are accustomed to regard him with well-founded suspicion'.

The faculty may also bear in mind the undesirability of having the curriculum planned by staff whose personal educational experiences have been more or less identical, and may take pains to appoint to the committee people who graduated from several different schools. While many opinions from many places undoubtedly ensure that all proposals are properly ventilated, they also ensure that there is plenty of scope for prolonged argument.

The result of these procedures is that discussions sometimes become acrimonious, and agreement difficult to reach. Furthermore, any decisions arrived at have to be referred to the faculty for approval, and on the faculty there are many people, with different sets of pre-judices, who suspect the reasoning and the motives behind the sug-gestions made by the committee. These are the people who, as Cornford points out, are prone to apply the epithet 'wild-cat' to a scheme 'unanimously agreed upon by experts after two years' exhaustive consideration of thirty-five or more alternative proposals'. They are counterbalanced by some of the more harassed senior teaching staff, whose minds are encumbered with so many other problems that they often approve a formidable new project without giving it the consideration that it requires. The minds of the junior faculty members, who may have the time for such consideration, usually lack the experience through which they can compare one project against another. As a consequence, public discussion of pro-posals for new departures in medical teaching is often disappointing; it is a case of 'si jeunesse savait, si vieillesse pouvait'. It is only after the consequences of its decisions sink in that the faculty has second thoughts, so that the matter is reopened and sent back to the com-mittee for reconsideration.

It is not surprising, therefore, that progress may be slow. In some schools discussion of curricular changes has proceeded for many years without appreciable results. An immense amount of time can be taken up in argument over this or that detail, time which often turns out eventually to have been totally unproductive. It is easy for a committee to become obsessed with a fancied need for change, and if half the energy that has been put into discussing new curricula in Britain since 1958 had been devoted to the actual job of teaching, many of the new curricular devices would have proved quite unnecessary.

The difficulty of securing an adequate body of agreement on the reforms to be instituted is less in schools headed by a strong character with a clear idea of what needs to be done—whether he is the dean or the chairman of the planning committee—since such characters may dominate the thinking of the faculty. But their views are not always to the liking of a substantial minority, and when their term of office expires, chaos may result.

New medical schools have an advantage when it comes to putting ideas together and securing their implementation, for they do not have to contend with the immense force of local tradition. In a school which has been in existence for many years, each department has its own individual foibles and beliefs. There are always traditionally minded 'diehards' among the staff, who are prepared to oppose any departure from the system which they are at present operating. Their objections most frequently take the form that their own particular 'subject' must be taught and examined in a certain way if it is not to become totally valueless. It is difficult to argue such points, since the professor of a subject has been appointed as the expert in this subject, and his word must be given due weight. The presence of one or two determined reactionaries may in fact wreck attempts at reorganization.

Secondly, new schools do not have to reckon with the difficulty presented by students already in the pipeline. During the period of transition an established medical school contains two sorts of students—those admitted under the old regulations, and those admitted under the new ones. Injustices may seem to be done to either group; for example, the new regulations may permit only two opportunities for the passing of a given examination, while the old regulations permit more. Or the old regulations may require a period of study of 6 years and the new ones a period of only 5. Such discrepancies cause a certain amount of ill-feeling among the students and among some of the staff, and require careful handling at the committee and faculty stages.

There are two ways of planning a curriculum for a new medical school. The unsatisfactory one is to appoint an outside planning committee before the school is actually founded. This committee may have no direct relationship with the new school, and may contain nobody who is to be appointed to the faculty, though it is common to include the dean-elect, if he is known. The other medical members are usually drawn from the ranks of the elder statesmen of the medical profession, and there may be several whose distinction is unquestioned, but whose experience of active teaching is very out-of-date. The findings of the committee may be published in a report, and the new faculty is expected to follow at least the outline of the recommendations. The predictable result of this procedure is that when the new staff are appointed they immediately set about altering the carefully framed regulations to conform with their own ideas.

The more satisfactory way of formulating a curriculum for a new medical school is to miss out this preliminary stage, which is inevitably superseded in any case, and to have the curriculum decided by some of those who are actually going to have to implement it. This means making the appointments to at least a number of key chairs well in advance of the date on which the school is to open its doors, so that the incumbents have plenty of time to discuss their own proposals. The committee so formed consists of the dean-elect, plus a small number of professors appointed at or about the same time; they are therefore usually in the same age-group, and nobody has academic seniority over anybody else, so that there are no 'father figures', crusted with authority and tradition, to be circumvented. Other members are drawn from the local medical profession and administration.

A small committee of this kind, operating on the spot under an understanding dean, has an excellent opportunity of getting to know the individual problems of its members, and of arguing about every conceivable matter over a series of quite informal meetings at which opinions can be freely expressed. If one participant thinks that something foolish is being proposed, he can there and then say so in round terms instead of retiring to his own department to brood over his wrongs. Under a system of this kind it is impossible for any foundation department represented to feel itself isolated from the course of events, and the paranoid reactions so common in established schools when a new curriculum is being planned can be almost completely avoided. Each head of department can be asked to submit his own concept of the content of the curriculum and the methods of teaching; he can then be asked to justify his proposals in front of the others—an ordeal reminiscent of a mediaeval disputation, for they can be encouraged to attack his most cherished ideas. Such experiences make the committee members think very seriously about whether their individual proposals are either valid or necessary.

Once the contributions of the individual departments are agreed, the attempt can be made to assemble them into a whole, and matters of method, timetabling, and logistics can be dealt with. Throughout all this period it is easy to maintain liaison between the members of the small group involved, and it is possible to preserve the initial impetus attached to doing something new, potentially valuable, and wholly exciting, even through a period of extremely hard work.

This idyllic situation naturally cannot last long. During the time of discussion new staff are constantly being appointed; some to new senior posts and others as juniors to the foundation members of the committee. With every new appointment the task of maintaining liaison becomes harder and harder, and, even though there are the best intentions of talking over every new proposal with the departmental staffs, the pressure of events and the rush of administrative detail tends to prevent this happening as often as it should. Some of the junior teaching staff, and indeed some of the in-coming professors, begin to think that they have been inadequately consulted on matters of policy, and to feel left out because they do not understand fully the reasons for various decisions and commitments. Liaison between the original senior appointees may continue to be excellent, but liaison between seniors and juniors, and between juniors in different departments, inevitably becomes less than perfect as the school grows. The price of unity is eternal communication, and this is difficult to maintain beyond a certain stage of growth.

It often happens that those involved in planning a new curriculum, either in a new or in an established school, retreat to their ivory towers again after 'completing' their task. Much of the advantage gained by their exploration of the points of view of their colleagues is thereby lost; the formulation of a new curriculum is not an end in itself, and those who make the plan are not entitled to feel that they have finished their work. They must continue to communicate among themselves, and also with the staffs of their departments. One of the commonest difficulties facing medical reformers is the reluctance of their committee members to embark on detailed explanations for every step taken. But the minutes of meetings at which decisions were arrived at are rarely of much use for communicating the sense behind the decisions, and explanatory meetings in every department, however tedious these may be, are essential.

To serve on a curriculum-planning committee, of whatever kind, is a profoundly educative experience. No one with any self-respect could spend his life teaching medicine without wishing that certain things were done better, and everyone has ideas regarding reform. In the modern permissive atmosphere surrounding medical education the committee members are apt to feel that they have a free hand to plan the millennium. They meet in an atmosphere of euphoria, and the room rapidly becomes filled with the buzz of the bees liberated from each individual bonnet.

The first chastening note in the hum of the swarm is the realization that the pattern of medical practice is changing at a very rapid rate. The products of a medical school are turned out into a world very different from that in which they began their studies, and, in spite of gallant attempts, such as those of Burnet (1964) and Ellis (1965), to prognosticate the needs of doctors and the state of medical practice in the future, a veil of pretty opaque uncertainty is, in the nature of things, likely to surround any deliberations the committee may embark upon. This induces a certain humility in some committee members, but, regrettably, not in all, and much effort may have to be expended in persuading some contributors to the discussions that they may not, after all, have found the key to the garden gate of the groves of Academe.

The speed of change in the outside world also means that the curriculum which is planned must be flexible enough to permit of alteration in response to modified conditions. The committee is therefore forced to realize that what it plans is a temporary measure only, and that its pet ideas may not survive longer than the first few years after the plan is put into operation. As soon as newcomers are brought in to teach or to learn in the school, the circumstances and opinions of these people must be taken into account, and the curriculum gradually modifies itself in accordance with the new material. In fact, changes in the curriculum may succeed each other with alarming rapidity once the initial decision to shake off the chains of tradition has been taken. This educational flux has the advantage that curricula rapidly evolve in different directions according to local circumstances, and so a basis is afforded on which natural selection can operate. The disadvantage is that, unless special care is taken to ensure the contrary, no scheme of action is in existence for long enough to allow it to be properly evaluated [see p. 178]. What is new is not necessarily better, and it is essential that the committee should know whether it is progressing in the right direction or in the wrong. This problem leads most committees to the ignominious conclusion that assessment of this kind is 'too difficult', and is simply set aside and ignored.

It is thus brought home to the committee member that he has embarked on the imposition of perhaps far-reaching changes which he will never be able to evaluate, and that his deliberations must necessarily be 'on a similar basis to the hunt for the philosopher's stone, with the added proviso that the stone will be unrecognizable even when it is found' (Sinclair, 1955).

The question which obviously arises in his mind after reaching this conclusion is, 'What are we doing all this *for*?' Only too often he receives no satisfactory answer, and sometimes he is brought to realize that much of what is proposed is based on nothing more than a desire to be 'with it', to remain in fashion. It has been well said: 'Never run after a bus, a woman, or an educational theory; there will be another one along in a minute.' Yet the fact remains that planning committees are willing, on the basis of the prejudices of their members, and without any factual data to go on, to reorganize the entire teaching programme—content as well as methods—without a clear statement of why they are trying to do it. I have actually heard it said by someone, 'Surely we all want to be as up-to-date as possible'. This is change for the sake of change, much like taking a motor-bicycle to pieces and trying to put it together again in a different way. 'Why?' is a question far too seldom heard in the deliberations of the committee.

Having learned all these lessons, but still pressing on with only slightly abated ardour, the committee member proceeds to encounter the practical difficulties of curricular change, and his enthusiasm rapidly becomes dampened by the realization that the 'free hand' he had supposed himself to possess is not quite so free as it appeared. No medical school exists in a vacuum (Sinclair, 1958), and the future is largely mapped out by the past.

For example, if the hospital is separated by too great a distance from the preclinical departments in the university campus, then transport difficulties may restrict close vertical collaboration. If funds are restricted, it is impossible to institute expensive methods of teaching, like the establishment of a full-blown tutorial system, which requires large numbers of staff. The general educational standard of the local school system may determine the teaching in the first year of the course. In places where biology is badly taught at the regional schools, it may be necessary to devote quite a little time to the teaching of biology to a satisfactory standard in the medical curriculum proper. If only a small percentage of entrants to the medical school have reached an advanced level of knowledge of chemistry in their Certificate of Education examinations, it is no good planning the curriculum on an assumption of this knowledge.

There is a relatively high failure rate in the early years of any university course, and the medical faculty is no exception. If the pattern of study is completely out of line with that obtaining in the faculty of science, medical students who find that they have made a mistake in their vocation, or who are unable to cope with one or more of the subjects in the medical course, may find it impossible to receive credit from the faculty of science for such successes as they may have achieved, and may have to start all over again at the beginning. Similarly, if the curriculum is radically different from medical curricula in other places, a considerable problem may arise over inter-university transfers, and this may cause hardship. For example, a student whose parents have gone to live in another part of the world may find it impracticable to stay in his present medical school, and may wish to accompany his family. If so doing means that he has to lose a year or two because the pattern of study he has been through does not fit with the curriculum of his new school, he is understandably upset.

There is also the problem of outside examinations and assessments. If a student's ability to earn his living by medical practice depends on his passing an outside examination, such as those of the National Boards in America, it is folly for a medical school to formulate a curriculum which will make it difficult for him to pass these examinations. This problem does not apply to the same extent in Britain, though it operates on those who wish to qualify by means of the Conjoint Board examinations [see p. 142].

All these and other difficulties may considerably sober the tyro planner, who may even come to react to his endeavours with a certain cynicism. Nevertheless, the enforced rethinking which discussions of this kind involve is of the greatest value to the teachers who take part in them. This is the best way of being compelled to consider one's teaching in relation to the work of others, and of coming to appreciate the problems of other departments. Too many medical teachers feel about their colleagues much as did Oscar Wilde: 'Other people are quite dreadful. The only possible society is oneself.' After a prolonged attempt to understand each other as members of a planning committee they may come to modify this opinion somewhat. 'Ignorance alone makes monsters or bugbears,' said Hazlitt, 'our actual acquaintances are all very commonplace people . . . we can scarcely hate anyone we know.'

At the same time most planning committees contain at least one empire builder, out to gain his own particular ends, even at the expense of other people's, and valuable experience may be gained in detecting and dealing with such special pleading.[1]

In spite of these humanizing influences, it is fatally easy for the

---

[1] 'He never wants anything but what's right and fair: only when you come to settle what's right and fair, it's everything that he wants and nothing that you want' (Hughes, *Tom Brown's Schooldays*).

MBE

committee member, whether new to the game or experienced, to become so involved in the mechanics of the curriculum—the examination schedules, the timetables, the arrangements for transport, the subdivision of teaching time into half-units and quarter-units—that he loses sight of the human side of the whole matter, the only side which really matters. He forgets the objectives which all these delicately interlocking arrangements are designed to further, and for this reason they must be regularly restated for his benefit.

IMPLEMENTATION AND CONTROL

No sooner have the regulations been settled and published and the first batch of student guinea-pigs started work than the programme which looked so perfect on paper proves to have unforeseen and unfortunate consequences. The class in mitochondrial behaviour is too big for the only available room, and it is necessary to move it to another spot in the timetable. The senior lecturer in bioactinics goes on past his time, so that the students cannot arrive in time for their tutorials in antisocial dimorphism. A new reader in orthonychia has been appointed, and the third-year curriculum, so laboriously assembled, has to be taken to pieces to accommodate the new speciality. The prevalence of anatomy oral examinations upsets the delicate susceptibilities of the physiologists and biochemists, whose subjects suffer from the distraction of attention. And so on; the list is inexhaustible.

This sort of problem is usually dealt with by appointing a curriculum committee, whose initial job it is to steer the new plan through the shallows of administrative difficulty, and to modify it and patch up its leaks so that it floats when thrown out into the smooth deep waters of routine. To determine the composition of this committee is in itself a matter of considerable difficulty. An attempt can be made to make it representative, in which case it becomes almost impossibly large, for to represent every department which has a hand in teaching a modern curriculum requires quite a considerable number of people. Or it can be made an elective body, in which case blocks of departments with similar hopes and fears can appoint someone to represent their point of view. Or it can be appointed by faculty on the basis of trying to secure the best people for the task. Obviously it must contain a wide spread of different disciplines ranging from the first to the final year of the curriculum, or else it would find it very difficult to do its job, and usually it has powers to co-opt in case it finds itself lacking expert advice when dealing with a particular problem. In every eventuality somebody somewhere is bound to feel some grievance, and may develop a paranoid reaction which sours general good relations. To be a member of a curriculum committee is not an easy assignment, and to be its chairman requires a reservoir of tact and persuasiveness if any sort of success is to be achieved.

Usually the curriculum committee finds it convenient to split up, for most day-to-day purposes, into smaller units, each of which may be given responsibility for a particular part of the curriculum. Thus, a subcommittee may be appointed to look after each academic year of the course, and to report back on its activities to the parent body at regular intervals. Only when problems arise between different years is the whole ponderous apparatus of the main curriculum committee invoked.

As in the planning committee, the chief difficulty is to avoid becoming entangled in administrative matters to such an extent that they obscure the importance of the attitudes of both teachers and taught. The committee must not allow details of timetabling, neatness of co-ordination, or splendour of assessment to supplant recognition of the human personalities and problems involved.

Indeed, this is an occupational risk shared by every member of the faculty. It is easy to become absorbed in the day-to-day running of the school; the students sit and pass examinations, they disappear from one department only to appear with clockwork precision in another, until finally there are no more departments for them to pass through, and the only thing is to give them a degree and let them go. The mere statement of this attitude is enough to expose its absurdity; one cannot mass-produce human lives as one can fabricate a motor-car. Yet this way of thinking, or something like it, is only too common in established medical schools where teaching has gone on for so long that the teachers have ceased to question what they are doing. It is therefore necessary from time to time to reiterate the objectives of the curriculum, and this duty ought to devolve on the curriculum committee in its capacity as guardian of the mysteries handed down by the planning committee.

At the risk of undue repetition, it is necessary to stress once more that from the earliest planning stage some provision for evaluation of the new curriculum should be built in, and this duty also should be entrusted to the curriculum committee. In an established medical school it is possible to put some sort of evaluation examination into the final-year assessment, so that adequate control data can be made available. While the new curriculum is working its way up from the first year, four or five cohorts of final-year students educated under the old dispensation can be assessed, unless changes are made in the intermediate years simultaneously with the implementation of the new first-year course. Even if this is done, two or three cohorts may still be assessable, and these will provide a baseline against which the performance of the 'guinea-pigs' can be tested.

In a new medical school it is much easier to design an evaluation programme, for it can be built into the routine assessment procedure instead of having to be added on top of it. But the difficulty is that there are no controls. However, it is certain that after a few years changes will develop in the curriculum, many of which are of such magnitude that it is desirable to evaluate their effect, and the new curriculum then becomes the control for its successors.

But there are other possibilities. It is not only desirable to compare the performances 'before' and 'after', but very worthwhile to attempt comparisons between different schools, some of which are operating an orthodox curriculum and some of which are trying experimental teaching. This can be done on the level of factual recall and understanding by an agreement among several schools to use the same examination papers simultaneously. This is difficult with essay questions, because of the variation in marking by different examiners, and some sort of 'blind' technique has to be used, three or four examiners each marking all the papers in ignorance of the source of the scripts, which are identified only by a code number. This is a big and tedious job, and it is certainly much easier to use multiple choice objective questions, which can be marked by machine, and which eliminate marking variation. It is possible to make use of the existing services of the National Board of Medical Examiners in America for this purpose, and to obtain from them a statement showing the position of the school in relation to the performance of other schools.[2] Or it is possible to devise a special examination designed to cover the objectives of the new programme and to allow comparison with other control schools who signify their willingness to take part (Saunders, 1967).

[2] The National Board organization has developed a 'Minitest' consisting of 360 pretested questions covering 12 'subject areas'. The questions, which are of the objective variety, are varied annually but the standard is kept constant, and the 'Minitest' is already in use in several American medical schools for the specific purpose of assessing curricular changes. A baseline is obtained by administering the test to the students entering upon the first year of the course, and they are then examined sequentially at the end of each year up to qualification (Jason, 1966; Levit, 1967).

It is true that so far other important matters such as clinical skill and student attitudes remain outside evaluation (Jacobson, 1967). But the patient management problems which have already been used for the purpose of evaluating the curriculum (Sinclair, 1972) are a big step in the direction of obtaining comparative data on clinical skill, and further development of psychological testing may allow us to examine student attitudes in the future. It is therefore important not to adopt a negative attitude towards evaluation, but to explore the possibilities by which some sort of meaningful assessment of curricular changes can be obtained.

PART THREE

General Review

9 Comments and Prognosis

Medical education is like religion in
that it can lead to a great deal of talk
with little useful action.

L. J. Witts

This is a restless age, when there is a tendency to think that what is
new is good and what is old is bad. Nobody has to prove this for it
to be accepted, for it is also a credulous and self-abasing age, when
people readily believe destructive criticism which is forcefully and
dogmatically put across, especially when it applies to institutions.
For some time now the whole concept of education in general, and
medical education in particular, has been in a state of flux, with new
methods of teaching flooding in every few years, or even months, to
displace the old ones—an old one being defined in this context as one
which has been in use for more than a year or two.

Because of the ball and chain applied to it by the General Medical
Council, British medical education took no part in the initial con-
vulsions which turned its American counterpart upside down just
after the last war, but it is now going through a phase in which
its practitioners are kicking up their heels in new-found freedom,
and there are few places in which reforming zeal has not gained a
foothold. Nevertheless, there are no new basic ideas, and most of
the innovations being tried out in this country are directly copied or
modified from the American experiments of the last 20 years or so.
The concepts underlying these ideas, though perfectly suitable for
application in their natural habitat, are often ill-adapted for
transplantation to a different ecological niche.

What our predecessors did was usually perfectly reasonable,
having regard to the conditions of the time. To sweep it away without a qualm, and to replace it with a completely untried system, is to
take a very considerable gamble, and a very arrogant one. Admittedly
change is necessary, but is revolution better than evolution? *Festina
lente* has always been a reasonable motto, and where the education

of the next generation is at stake it is perhaps particularly necessary to exercise caution.

But in a society in which 'permissiveness' and 'freedom from constraint' have been elevated to the status of all-important objectives it is difficult to resist 'liberalization' of education without being labelled as reactionary. No one is quite so sure of the virtue of his own ideas as an intellectual mounted on his hobby-horse, and to call them in question is to invite emotional abuse. This is perhaps not unexpected among politicians or economists, but it is surely a negation of everything that science and medicine stand for that curricular reforms have virtually no basis in factual evidence. As Ashby (1963) said, of British academics in general, 'All over the country these groups of scholars, who would not make a decision about the shape of a leaf or the derivation of a word or the author of a manuscript without painstakingly assembling the evidence, make decisions about admissions policy, size of universities, staff-student ratios, content of courses, and similar issues, based on dubious assumptions, scrappy data and mere hunch'.

Again, once a scheme has been decided upon, it would seem obvious that it should be allowed time to prove itself. But only too often changes are made which are superseded by further alterations after an interval of a few months, and when these prove momentarily difficult to operate, a new and contradictory system is introduced to rectify matters. There is a well-known definition of a zealot as someone who redoubles his efforts when he has lost sight of his aim, and this definition applies with some force to many educational reformers, for whom change becomes a desirable end in itself, without reference to the objectives which this change is supposed to be promoting. The most serious consequence of this attitude is that none of the changes made gets even the most superficial evaluation before it is succeeded by another one, usually on the basis of administrative convenience.

British students are nowadays subjected to a heavy and increasing load of science-based teaching. The need for a thorough grounding in the scientific aspects of medicine is stressed because the medicine of the future is apparently to be completely scientific. But there is an unspoken fallacy in this argument (Platt, 1967; Illingworth, 1968), for it implies that nobody can make use of a scientific discovery unless he thoroughly understands the theory on which it is based, and something of the experimental work by which this theory was arrived at. In everyday life this is, of course, nonsense. The housewife who switches on the television set is making use of an extremely complicated electronic apparatus, and may be totally ignorant of how it works, yet she knows what knob to turn to produce a given effect. But it is argued that a doctor cannot diagnose and treat a cut hand unless he is well versed in the biochemical and cellular processes of growth and repair, and has personally examined electron micrographs of collagen fibres. How many doctors who daily, and successfully, prescribe propanolol or nitrazepam know anything about their chemical structure and degradation products? There is coming to be too much emphasis on hard science in medical education, and too little on the practical and empirical side of life. This is, of course, the swing of the pendulum, but it is perhaps time that it was given a little nudge in the opposite direction again.[1] The danger is that the increasing influence of science over the conduct of the medical course will force the human aspects of both teaching and doctoring into the background. This, for me, would be a tragedy, and I think I speak for most patients throughout the world. And if it is argued that a good grounding in sociology and psychology is a satisfactory substitute for the personal approach, the kindliness inculcated by example, the charity, in the biblical sense of the word, and the understanding, of the doctor-patient relationship, my reply is a resounding negative. This is the thing, above all, that we are in danger of losing under the new dispensation, and may have already lost. Already patients are being diagnosed by computer, examined by technicians, and treated by impersonal underlings. Is this what we want for the future? We are stumbling into a new age without even considering where we are going, changing our educational policy at the dictates of fashion, making no attempt to chart our path or to find out where we are when we get there.

The present ascendancy of science depends to a major extent on the staffing difficulties of the preclinical departments [see p. 43] which excite minimal attention among medical educators and clinicians, but are a basic determinant of the whole 'set' of medical education in the future. The plight of the clinical departments, whose staff will shortly have to take much wider responsibility for the postgraduate education of a much larger number of graduates, is certainly talked about, but the full implications of the situation do not seem to have sunk in, or to have been considered in terms of the effort necessarily diverted away from undergraduate teaching.

For Henry Miller (1971) the villain who 'resists the liberalizing of

---

[1] 'Science is throughout the servant, not the master, a servant to be used with understanding and called on unsparingly in the patient's interest, but dismissed peremptorily and without remorse on all those many occasions when the patient is better off without its services.' (Platt, 1967.)

the Royal Commission' is the preclinician, who has achieved a 'stranglehold' on the curriculum, but there are many preclinicians, perhaps particularly in London, who would reply to this that pots are in no position to call kettles black. Some clinicians have in the past been pretty outspoken in their condemnation of their colleagues in the earlier phases of medical education, and from the literature one might suppose that everything in the clinical garden is lovely. One has only to ask any medical student in any medical school to find out that this is very far from the truth (Sinclair, 1957b), and one is led to suspect that the clinical teachers believe that attack is the best form of defence.

We are all in the same glass house and it does little good to anyone to throw stones. We should rather be concerned in a corporate effort to patch up the existing holes in the fabric as best we can. But the differences of opinion are symptomatic of a progressive divergence of interests, partly real and partly fancied, between those who teach in the earlier part of the curriculum and those whose contribution is made later.

Miller (1971) has 'grave doubts about the continued viability of the isolated preclinical phase of medical education. . . . The pure morphologist and the academic physiologist will gravitate to faculties of science, the anatomy and physiology relevant to medicine being taught throughout the whole of a clinically oriented course by clinicians and scientists in collaboration'. As he points out, problems of recruitment are more likely to effect such a change than deliberate academic decisions.

The Royal Commission does not seem to have understood this point. On the one hand they recommend that there should be as much integration of preclinical and clinical teaching as possible, and on the other they advise a course structure (3 years of science-based preclinical teaching followed by a science degree) which, taken in conjunction with the declining medical interest in preclinical teaching as a career, seems certain to cut off preclinical from clinical teaching as effectively as could be wished.

Perhaps it might do us good, and help us to see things in perspective, if we turned for a time from our obsession with the curriculum to consider the students and teachers who take part in it. For example, a most important advance would be effected if all staff who take part in teaching could be persuaded that teaching is just as important as research, and that just as much effort should be put into it. This proposition is quite strange to many of them, since from their point of view it seems obvious that the university is not interested in the standard of teaching, though it is very keen on research. Every year it demands a statement of research publications, and these are combined together and published as representing the work of the university. Admittedly it is difficult to quantify teaching and impossible to estimate the value of individual contributions to it [see p. 159], but the whole atmosphere suggests to the junior teacher (and to many of his seniors) that the only important thing is to accumulate as many respectable publications as possible in the shortest possible time. This, and this alone, appears to them as the road by which they can reach promotion and eventually control what is (sometimes rather inappropriately) called a 'teaching department'.

Many junior teachers enjoy talking about teaching methods and new curricular programmes, but are understandably lost when it comes to the actual teaching required. Teaching is not an easy art, and has to be learned. With the learning may come a loss of the initial enthusiasm; it is never so exciting to implement a new curriculum as it is to plan it, and when the extraordinary has become the commonplace the pioneer spirit may dissipate completely. For this reason many promising schemes degenerate, the spirit being replaced by the letter of the (by now) mechanical routine. If some means could only be devised of keeping the initial atmosphere of co-operation and interest in existence, it would have an incalculable effect on the future of British medical education.

The lack of maturity of British students in the early part of their course is a fundamental factor which receives much less than its due attention. The Hale Report (1964) suggested the possibility of having the Certificate of Education examinations for schoolchildren in the autumn and postponing the start of the university year until the following January; this would allow university entrants a little additional time, free from further study, in which to grow up. This is not a new idea. Marshall (1951), talking of the entrance qualifications of American medical students, suggested that 'medical schools might better demand a certificate that at least one year had been spent no closer than five miles to a college campus.' Winston Churchill put it rather differently: 'It is only when they are really thirsty for knowledge, longing to hear about things, that I would let them go to the University. It would be a favour, a coveted privilege, only to be given to those who had either proved their worth in factory or field or whose qualities and zeal were pre-eminent.' That British students would benefit from an interval between leaving school and entering university seems undeniable; one has only to remember the keenness and enthusiasm of the medical students returning after the war. But here we are brought back once more to the financial side of things; neither the country, it is claimed, nor the individual, can afford such an interval.

But we can, and should, think seriously about the entrance qualifications we prescribe. Pickering (1968) sets his sights high: 'I hope that we shall all work to admit into the University course for Medicine boys and girls who are educated citizens, that is to say, who can speak and write their own language lucidly and grammatically, who are familiar with mathematics, I would say, to Calculus level, who can speak and read a little in two foreign languages, preferably living, who are interested in art and literature and current affairs, and who know the elements of science.' He adds, 'This may seem a lot, but it is no more than was common enough among the entrants to medicine when I was young'. *O tempora! O mores!* I should like to side with Pickering, but my native pessimism leads me to settle for the criterion cited by Dorst (1947): 'I would be happy if the students who came to me could only read and write English and know what it means.' It is just possible that the present state of flux in secondary education may eventually provide for this possibility, but for the moment pessimism seems the only logical reaction.

But if this sort of thing is what we want, why do we not go after it? For years those engaged in medical education have been saying something similar and behaving quite differently. The secondary schools have observed our lip service to a general education and our rigid insistence in practice on science as the only prerequisite we are prepared to recognize, and their attitude can be summed up in the words of the slip with which miswritten cheques are returned: 'Words and figures do not agree.' Even the Royal Commission envisages that most candidates will continue to offer three A-level science subjects in the General Certificate of Education because, it is said, of the demands of biochemistry and physiology. But if we feel strongly enough about the blinkered minds of some of our entrants, cut off from the sights and sounds around them, could we not, perhaps, consider modifying the demands of biochemistry and physiology? Industry now seems to accept a university degree, in whatever subject, as a certificate of general competence rather than an indication of specialized ability: people with first-class honours in zoology run computer services, and physicists become personnel managers. Is it not possible to adopt a little of this spirit, and to accept a suitably balanced Certificate of Education as an indication of general academic capacity? As Wyman (1971) has said: 'The physics, chemistry and biology of my day bear little resemblance to that

taught today. How important is it then to have such a detailed knowledge of a few scientific subjects which can apparently only be obtained
by the sacrifice of a general education, when love of the English language and appreciation of English literature, history and the arts do not
alter with time. . . . So many consultants tell me that their housemen,
at the end of a lengthy education, are still unable to write a lucid case-
history and many of them still have difficulty with elementary spelling.'

Having admitted our candidates, should we not make every effort
to help them over the troublesome transition to the university?
Should we not, for example, try a little remedial therapy by showing
them how to learn? The schools do not, apparently, undertake this,
and so many students have difficulties in this direction that some form
of help is obviously necessary, though nobody seems to regard it as
his business. Then again, are we quite sure that when speaking
to junior students we try to express our ideas and requirements
in the simplest possible manner? The profession of medicine has
become completely overrun by jargon, and words take the place
of ideas. The students who learn from us pick up the jargon, which is
powerful magic, and lose the ideas behind it. The Royal Society
wished to exact from its members 'a close, naked, natural way of
speaking, positive expressions, clear senses, a native easiness, bringing all things as near the mathematical plainness as they can'. We
cannot all do this, but we can all try; the student's task would be
much easier if we did.

And when we come to assess the talents, intelligence, and particular aptitudes of the students we have been teaching, are we to be
satisfied to have it done for us by a machine? Underlying every
teaching activity ought to be the principle enunciated by Pickering
(1959) that 'whatever else we do, we should be absolutely sure that
each of us, when he has finished, leaves the student with a finer mind
than when he started'. The yardstick by which Pickering (and I)
would like to measure success in this direction is at present completely
out of fashion and apparently regarded with something akin to
contempt: 'Perhaps the surest guide . . . is the student's ability to
express himself lucidly, accurately, and grammatically, his ability to
marshal his evidence and draw his conclusions.' The swing of assessment techniques towards objective examinations is part of the swing
towards science rather than medicine; electrons have a hypnotic
fascination, and anything that is discovered by their use is often
thought of as in some way superior to things that depend on more
mundane pieces of apparatus, such as the human mind. There is no
question but that they are superior to essay questions in terms of

convenience, and I am prepared to make a virtue out of necessity by acquiescing in their use, but nothing more.

It may be that in the future this is the only kind of qualifying examination we shall use, for in the European Economic Community an agreed form of outside assessment may well have to be instituted [see p. 142], and this would almost inevitably be of objective type. This examination might also replace the final examinations set by the individual schools, much as the National Board examinations in America are taken by nearly everybody, for the licence to practise may be made dependent on passing it. We may not be as far away from the 'one portal of entry' to the medical profession as we think, and this portal may turn out to be of such a character as to dispense with the ability to write English.

Whatever the objective examination can do for us, it cannot evaluate the character of the candidates; yet this is one of the most important factors in their future careers. There have been several attempts to define the character and accomplishments of the ideal 'basic doctor', and every one of us has, no doubt, his own mental image of such a man. I have put character first, because, in the prevailing atmosphere of science-based education, this aspect of the matter often goes by default. We have no real idea of the character of the individuals we herd together in our mass-production classes until it is too late to do much about it, and the way in which they develop during the course may or may not contribute towards the desirable image we have in mind. Character-building has always been considered a worthy objective in British secondary schools, but in the universities we confine ourselves to hoping that the job will be done for us by the students themselves. It is, however, a good sign that student counselling services are growing up in most universities, and that several have regent schemes whereby the student can obtain advice on personal problems or other non-academic difficulties.

The changes in the medical curriculum—it is a contradiction in terms to call them experiments (Sinclair, 1955)—which are at present in progress have cost the medical schools an enormous total of man-hours of discussion; agenda and minutes pile up mountains of prolixity;[2] reports and pamphlets, surveys and statistics proliferate like rabbits; administrators and student advisers, course integrators and committee chairmen are appointed and resign; students are questioned and their opinion is canvassed at faculty meetings and staff/student committees. And what is it all for? Shall we be better at the end of it? Perhaps, for a time. The endless talk and argument

[2] 'Revolutions,' as Leon Trotsky said, 'are always verbose.'

do at least inform those with minds open enough to be informed that education is a difficult and chancy business, and that other people have problems just as pressing as their own. When the excitement dies down, we shall certainly be told, like little Peterkin, that 'twas a famous victory. But as a new generation of teachers enters the medical faculties, many of them scientists rather than doctors, and interested in research and publication rather than in the quality of a profession not primarily their own, the situation will change again. These people will not have had the experience of planning and the exchange of ideas with other teachers of very different subjects; they will be experts in their own fields rather than admirable Crichtons, and their objectives will be to see that their own particular subjects are properly taught. The association of feudal states [see p. 75] will once more revert to bickering over the sharing out of the timetable, and in another 20 years or so a new call for reform will emerge, to meet conditions of practice so different from those of today and tomorrow that we cannot even guess at them. I should like to support Brotherston (1962) who deplores the possibility that we should revert to 'a kind of all or nothing technique of a new curriculum every 25 years and nothing in between'. As he rightly says, what is needed is 'continuing discussion and self-criticism of our teaching, not in an atmosphere of periodic frenzy, but as an organized and quietly sustained exercise'.

Abstractions, in the hands of university teachers, are always good for a solid 3 or 4 hours of debate at a time, and the education of a doctor is a topic full of abstractions. But there is a limit to conversation of this kind, and if it is carried on at the expense of the proper vocation of the participants it becomes a bad thing. Until 1957 the General Medical Council left no room for manoeuvre; the freedom since then has perhaps left too much. We have had 14 years in which to explore our own ideas, and although this has been a most healthy period of discussion, which has broadened the outlook of most members of medical faculties, some of them have now reached a stage where they might perhaps be prepared to welcome back a degree of benevolent dictatorship; it is always pleasant to have something to grumble about. There is a well-known Chinese curse which says, 'May you live in interesting times'. We have been doing just this, and for some of us it is becoming a little bit wearing. Surely the time is now ripe to let things be for a brief period in which attention can be turned to other matters of equal or greater importance, such as establishing personal contact with the students who will succeed us, advancing our subjects, and in general fulfilling our role as members of the most important profession in the world—that of teacher.

NBE

Appendix: Organization of Teaching

A. INTEGRATION

TABLE 2 summarizes the programme in Western Reserve University School of Medicine in 1958. It consists of three phases spread over 4 years' instruction, and includes several features—a preceptor (tutorial) system, the use of electives, free time, and projects—not directly relevant to the integration of study, but contributing to the distinctiveness of the curriculum. Other features, such as the initial orientation programme, the multidiscipline laboratories, and the scheme whereby students visited obstetrical patients and their families at home, are not shown. The programme in 1958 was substantially different from the programme with which the system was instituted in 1952, as a result of the progressive reassessment of teaching and learning undertaken by the faculty.

TABLE 2
WESTERN RESERVE UNIVERSITY
School of Medicine

PHASE 1 Normal Biology of Man		PHASE 2 Principles of Medicine			PHASE 3 Clinical Medicine		OBJECTIVE
	Projects 1 day / week	Phase 2A	Projects 1 day / week	Phase 2B	Bioclinical study sections	Thesis	
Cell biology*	Anatomy on infant cadaver	Introduction to disease	Anatomy on adult cadaver (three semesters)	Locomotor system	Required	Months	Scientific method
Tissue biology		Infectious disease		Nervous system	Basic clerkship	4	
neuro-muscular		Chemical agents		Ophthalmology	Medicine or Pediatrics		Biologic and clinical sciences
Cardiovascular		Cardiovascular disease		Female genital disease	Ambulatory clerkship	2	
respiratory		Respiratory		Endocrine, metabolic disease	Group clinic		
Metabolism		Hemopoietic			Obstetrics and gynecology	2	
Endocrine		Gastro-intestinal system		Legal medicine, psychiatry 1 hour per week	Basic surgical clerkship	2	
Correlation and review		Urinary disease			(Vacation)	2	
*Biostatistics		Male genitalia					
Introduction to library first three weeks		Skin					
Preceptor No. 1 Infant and family		Preceptor Nos. 2, 3 Clinical method			Preceptor No. 4 Continuity Program		Thinking as a physician
		Free Time One and one-half week days are free			Electives — Clinical, Teaching, Research, Biologic science — 4 months		Self-education
First Year		Second Year	Third Year		Fourth Year		

Source: Boake, W. C., and Epstein, I. S. (1958) Medical education at Western Reserve University, Cleveland, Med. J. Aust., 1, 280–2.

In Phase 1 the various tissues and organs of the body were studied systematically, structure and function being presented synchronously, and co-ordinated both with the process of dissection of a stillborn infant and with instruction in the methods of clinical examination. In Phase 2 there was 'system' integration (morbid anatomy, pathological physiology and biochemistry, pharmacology and therapeutics) co-ordinated with the anatomy of the adult cadaver. Phase 3 was mainly clinical, and included electives and the presentation of a thesis based on the project work undertaken throughout the course.

TABLE 3 gives an example (from proposals made by the University of Glasgow in 1962) of the way in which material relevant to a particular system can be combined and presented, and TABLE 4 shows how a portion of this programme may be timetabled.

TABLE 3
CONTENT OF TEACHING ON THE CARDIOVASCULAR SYSTEM

Medicine lectures (50 min.)
Causes of heart disease
Cardiac failure
Treatment of cardiac failure
Arrhythmias
Common types of congenital heart disease
Acute rheumatic infection and subacute
   bacterial endocarditis
Rheumatic heart disease
Types of and investigation of ischaemic
   heart disease
Treatment of ischaemic heart disease
Peripheral vascular disease
Forms of hypertension
Management of hypertension
Cor pulmonale; thyrotoxic heart disease

Symposia (1½ hours + discussion)
Anatomy, Histology, Physiology
'Cardiac muscle and conducting system'
(including electrophysiology and theory
of unipolar leads)

Physiology, Medicine, Surgery
'Methods of investigation and treatment
of congenital heart disease'

Pathology, Biochemistry, Medicine
'Atherosclerosis'

Pathology, Medicine, Radiology
'Aetiology and investigation of cases of
hypertension'

Anatomy lectures (40 min.)
  The normal heart (including radiology)
  Embryology of normal heart with theories
    of developmental abnormalities
  Anatomy of circulation, including coronary
    arteries
  Innervation of vessels and anatomy of
    sympathectomy

Clinico-Pathological conferences (40 min.)
Physician and Pathologist
  Cardiac failure
  Congenital heart disease
  Ischaemic heart disease
  Hypertension

Lecture demonstrations (40 min.)
  Arrhythmias
  ECGs normal and arrhythmias
  Rheumatic heart disease—ECGs and
    X-rays
  ECGs in ischaemic heart disease
  ECGs in hypertension
  Radiology in ischaemic disease

Pathology lectures (50 min.)
  Cardiac failure
  Rheumatic heart disease
  Ischaemic heart disease
  Hypertension

Panel discussions (50 min.)
Aftercare of young cardiac invalids—
Physician, Almoner, GP

Surgery of acquired heart disease
  (with film)   Surgeon
                    Physician

Surgery of vascular disease
                    Surgeon
                    Physician

Question session
                    Surgeon
                    Physician
                    Pathologist

Treatment of arrhythmias
                    Physician
                    Member of Materia
                    Medica Staff

Surgical lectures (50 min.)
Surgery of coronary disease
Films:
Surgery of acquired heart disease
Surgery of coronary heart disease

Displays:
Pathology Cardiac failure
           Bacteriology of heart disease
           Pathology of ischaemic heart
             disease
           Pathology of hypertensive
             disease
ECGs   Normals and arrhythmias
           ECGs of congenital heart
             disease and mitral stenosis
           Of ischaemic heart disease
           Hypertensive heart disease
X-rays   Congenital and acquired
             heart disease
           Hypertensive disease

TABLE 4
CARDIOVASCULAR SYSTEM: WEEK 3

TIME	MONDAY	TUESDAY	WEDNESDAY	THURSDAY	FRIDAY
9–11 a.m.	Clinics	Clinics	Clinics	Clinics	Clinics
11.15–12 noon	Autopsy	*Anatomy lecture* Anatomy of circulation, including coronary arteries	*Lecture/Demonstration* ECG in ischaemic heart disease	Autopsy	*CPC* Ischaemic heart disease
12 noon–1 p.m.	*Medical lecture* Ischaemic heart disease—types and investigation	*Biochemistry lecture*	*Medical lecture* Ischaemic heart disease—treatment	*Lecture and film* Surgery of coronary disease	*Medical lecture* Peripheral vascular disease
2–3 p.m.	Free Time	*Symposium:* Pathologist Biochemist Physician 'Atherosclerosis'	Free Time	Biochemistry Practical Work	Free Time
3–5 p.m.	*Pathology lecture* Ischaemic heart disease		Free Time	Biochemistry Practical Work	*Lecture/Demonstration* X-rays in ischaemic heart disease

Displays available all week: ECGs of ischaemic heart disease and pathology of ischaemic heart disease.

Source: Flemming, C. M. (1962) The new medical curriculum in the University of Glasgow, *Scot. med. J.*, **7**, 333–40.

B. CO-ORDINATION

TABLE 5 shows the second-year co-ordinated programme in the University of Western Australia in 1960. In the third year (not shown) the departments of anatomy, physiology and biochemistry took part in combined teaching with the clinical departments. The head and neck were dissected, and an examination of the anatomy of the central nervous system and the special senses was co-ordinated with the physiology of the nervous system and with a course in psychology. The department of anatomy collaborated with that of paediatrics in a course on post-natal growth and development, and the department of physiology combined with that of pathology to discuss disturbances of normal function.

TABLE 5
SECOND-YEAR PROGRAMME

TERM / TOPOGRAPHICAL ANATOMY	GENERAL ANATOMY AND HISTOLOGY	FUNCTIONAL AND CLINICAL ASPECTS STRESSED	GROWTH	PHYSIOLOGY	BIOCHEMISTRY
1. Upper extremity	Locomotor system; peripheral nerve; epithelia; tissues. General account of nervous system and its histology. Components of brain and cord. Autonomic system.	Fractures; dislocations; nerve injuries; life history and cancer of breast; movements of hand and digits; infections of hand. Injection sites. Radiology. Surface anatomy. Reflexes, plexuses, sensory and motor systems; general control of other systems. Clinical examination of CNS.	Radiology of limb at different ages. Brief account of development from simple tube.	Cell potentials; muscle; nerve. Autonomic system.	Biocatalysis; glycolysis; Krebs'cycle; muscle fatigue. Nervous tissue.
2. (a) Lower extremity	Blood:—counts; films; life history of formed elements.	Fractures; dislocations; nerve injuries. Locking mechanisms of joints; flat feet; standing, walking. Femoral hernia. Injection sites. Radiology. Surface anatomy.	Radiology of limb at different ages.	Blood; tissue fluid.	Blood; tissue fluid. Protein metabolism.
(b) Thorax	Cardiovascular system; lymphatics. Respiratory system.	Anatomy and functions of nose; anatomy of speech. Segments respiratory movements. Anatomy of lungs; tuberculosis. Coronary circulation. Clinical examination of chest. Surface anatomy.	Foetal circulation; changes at birth.	Cardiovascular system; respiration.	Blood; respiration
(c) Abdominal Wall	Anatomy of secretion; exocrine glands. Alimentary tract to stomach.	Anatomy of swallowing. Descent of testis. Inguinal and umbilical herniae.		Cardiovascular system; respiration.	Blood; respiration
3. Abdomen and pelvis	Alimentary and urogenital systems. Spermatogenesis; oogenesis. Endocrine glands.	Anatomy of peristalsis, defaecation and micturition. Appendicitis; perforated ulcer; pelvic floor. Surface and rectal examination. Clinical investigation of abdomen. Radiology.	Rotation of gut to explain adult relationships.	Alimentary system; excretion; endocrines.	Digestion; food transport; excretion; metabolism. Endocrines.

Source: Sinclair, D. C. (1965*b*) Preclinical teaching programme in the faculty of Medicine, University of Western Australia, *Indian J. med. Educ.*, **5**, 1–10.

TABLE 6 shows an integrated essay-type examination of the kind which followed the second-year programme. It was supplemented by an oral examination in which the student was confronted simultaneously by representatives of all three preclinical departments. At the end of the third year the separate examinations in each preclinical subject contained clinically oriented questions, and clinicians took part as examiners.

TABLE 6

SPECIMEN PAPER

HUMAN BIOLOGY

PAPER I

(Second-Year Medical Students)

Time allowed—*three* hours.

Four questions to be answered.

> Students are expected to integrate their anatomical, physiological and biochemical knowledge in answering each of the questions.

1. Describe the structure of the unit of kidney function (the nephron), and discuss how the glomerular filtrate is progressively modified into urine.

2. Discuss the composition and functions of the gastric juice. How, and by what structures, are its constituents formed?

3. Discuss the changes which take place in a voluntary muscle fibre during and after a single contraction. How is the arrangement of fibres in a voluntary muscle related to the functions of the muscle?

4. Give an account of the growth of a long bone. What are the physiological and biochemical processes concerned?

TABLE 6 *continued*

5. Discuss the part played by Insulin in the stabilization of the blood sugar level. Describe the structures which elaborate the hormone and the physiological processes which control its rate of production.

Source: Sinclair, D. C. (1965*b*) Preclinical teaching programme in the faculty of medicine, University of Western Australia, *Indian J. med. Educ.,* **5,** 1–10.

References

ACHESON, E. D. (1969) Medical school at Southampton, *Brit. med. J.*, **2**, 750–2.

ALLEN, M. (1969) Quality of medical education, *Brit. med. J.*, **2**, 528.

'A MEDICAL STUDENT' (1890) '*A Letter to Edinburgh Professors*': *Edited, with Preface, by a Graduate of Eminence*, London.

AMOS, S., DUNCAN, C. J., GILDER, R. S., HALL, R., and SMART, G. A. (1969) Tape-slide programmes in medical education at the university of Newcastle upon Tyne, *Brit. J. med. Educ.*, **3**, 362–8.

ANDERSON, J. (1966) Medical education and social change, in *The Evolution of Medical Education in Britain*, ed. Poynter, F. N. L., London.

ANDERSON, J., and ROBERTS, F. J. (1965) *A New Look at Medical Education*, London.

ARING, C. D. (1958) The medical uses of literacy, *Perspect. Biol. Med.*, **1**, 439–46.

ARNOTT, W. M. (1949) Reform in medical education, *Brit. med. J.*, **2**, 497–502.

ASHBY, E. (1963) Decision-making in the academic world, in *Sociological Studies in British University Education*, Monograph No. 7, The Sociological Review, University of Keele, Keele.

ASHBY, E., and ANDERSON, M. (1970) *The Boundaries of Student Participation*, London.

ATLAY, J. B. (1903) *Sir Henry Wentworth Acland*, London.

BADENOCH, J. (1967) The tutorial system at Oxford, *Brit. J. med. Educ.*, **1**, 108–10.

BARABAS, A. (1965) Blackboard drawing in medical teaching, *Brit. med. J.*, **1**, 782–4.

BARZUN, J. (1959) *The House of Intellect*, New York.

BEARD, R. M. (1969) A conspectus of research and development, in *Assessment of Undergraduate Performance*, Report of Conference at the University of London convened by the Committee of Vice-Chancellors and Principals and the Association of University Teachers, 27 March, London.

BEARD, R. M. (1970) *Teaching and Learning in Higher Education*, Harmondsworth.

BECKER, H. S., and GEER, B. (1958a) The fate of idealism in medical school, *Amer. sociol. Rev.*, **23**, 50–6.

BECKER, H. S., and GEER, B. (1958b) Student culture in medical school, *Harvard Educational Review*, **28**, 70–80.

BENDER, R. M. (1969) Attitudes toward grading systems used in medical education, *J. med. Educ.*, **44**, 1076–81.

BERRY, G. P. (1953) Medical education in transition, *J. med. Educ.*, **28**, 17–42.

BIBBY, J. (1970) Rewards and careers, *Higher Educ. Rev.*, **3**, 9–18.

BIRAN, L. A., and PICKERING, E. (1968) Unscrambling a herringbone; an experimental evaluation of branching programming, *Brit. J. med. Educ.*, **2**, 213–19.

BLAUG, M. (1968) The productivity of universities, in *Universities and Productivity*, Conference convened through the Joint Consultative Committee of the Vice-Chancellors' Committee and the Association of University Teachers, London.

BLIGH, D. A. (1970) The case for a variety of teaching methods in each lesson, *Brit. med. J.*, **4**, 202–9.

BOAKE, W. C., and EPSTEIN, I. S. (1958) Medical education at Western Reserve University, Cleveland, *Med. J. Aust.*, **1**, 280–2.

BRIDGES, P. (1970) Paper presented at meeting of British Association, London.

BRITISH JOURNAL OF MEDICAL EDUCATION (1969) The management of the medical school, *Brit. J. med. Educ.*, **3**, 168–9.

BRITISH MEDICAL ASSOCIATION (1948) *The Training of a Doctor*, London.

BRITISH MEDICAL JOURNAL (1968) Early exit, Editorial, *Brit. med. J.*, **3**, 390.

BRITISH MEDICAL STUDENTS' ASSOCIATION (1956) *First Report of the Subcommittee of the British Medical Students' Association on Undergraduate Medical Education in Great Britain and Northern Ireland*, British Medical Students' Association, London

BRITISH MEDICAL STUDENTS' ASSOCIATION (1957) *Second Report of the Subcommittee of the British Medical Students' Association on Undergraduate Medical Education in Great Britain and Northern Ireland*, British Medical Students' Association, London.

BROOK, G. L. (1968) The functions of the university teacher, in *Universities and Productivity*, Conference convened through the Joint Consultative Committee of the Vice-Chancellors' Committee and the Association of University Teachers, London.

BROOKE, B. N. (1970) Audiovisual aids in medical schools, *Lancet*, ii, 817–18.

BROTHERSTON, J. H. F. (1962) The new curricula, *Scot. med. J.*, **7**, 291–5.

BROTHERSTON, J. H. F., MARTIN, F. M., and BODDY, F. A. (1963) *Interim Report of the Medical Student Enquiry*, Association for the Study of Medical Education, London.

BUCKLEY-SHARP, M. D., and HARRIS, F. T. C. (1970) The banking of multiple-choice questions, *Brit. J. med. Educ.*, **4**, 42–52.

BULL, G. M. (1956) An examination of the final examination in medicine, *Lancet*, **ii**, 368–72.

BURNET, M. (1964) Fifty years on, *Brit. med. J.*, **2**, 1091–3.

BURNET, M. (1971) *Genes, Dreams and Realities*, Aylesbury.

BURY, R. de (1345) *Philobiblon*, Text and translation of E. C. Thomas, ed. Maclagan, M., Limited edition published 1960, Oxford.

CAMPBELL, E. J. M. (1970) The McMaster medical school at Hamilton, Ontario, *Lancet*, ii, 763–7.

CANTRELL, E. G., and CRAVEN, J. L. (1969) A trial of television in teaching clinical medicine, *Brit. J. med. Educ.*, 3, 110–14.

CAUGHEY, F. L. (1956) Western Reserve: clinical teaching during four years, *J. med. Educ.*, 31, 530–4.

CHANCE, R. A., and HUMPHRIES, D. A. (1966) Medical students' powers of observation, *Brit. J. med. Educ.*, 1, 131–4.

CHARVAT, J., MCGUIRE, C., and PARSONS, V. (1968) *A Review of the Nature and Uses of Examinations in Medical Education*, World Health Organization, Geneva.

CHRISTIE, R.V. (1969) Medical education and the State, *Brit. med. J.*, 2, 385–90.

CLARKE, E. (1966) History of British medical education, *Brit. J. med. Educ.*, 1, 7–15.

CLAXTON, E. E., and QUILLIAM, T. A. (1968) Essential evaluation criteria for medical films and videotape, in *Communication Media in Medicine*, B.I.S.F.A., London.

COHEN, H. (1950) Methods and men in the teaching of clinical medicine, *Brit. med. J.*, 2, 478–81.

COHEN, H. (1968) Medical education in Great Britain and Ireland, 1858–1967, *Brit. J. med. Educ.*, 2, 87–97.

COHEN, R. D., HUGHES, D. T. D., and RICHARDSON, P. C. (1957) Medical students look West: impressions of some American medical schools, *Lancet*, ii, 407–9.

COLTON, T., and PETERSON, O. L. (1967) An assay of medical students' abilities by oral examination, *J. med. Educ.*, 42, 1005–14.

COLWILL, J. M. (1969) Free time in the medical curriculum, *J. med. Educ.*, 44, 510–14.

CORNFORD, F. (1908) *Microcosmographia Academica* (6th ed. reprinted 1966), London.

COWLES, J. T. (1954) Current trends in examination procedures, *J. Amer. med. Ass.*, 155, 1383–7.

COWLES, J. T. (1965) A critical-comments approach to the rating of medical students' clinical performance, *J. med. Educ.*, 40, 188–98.

COX, R. (1967) Examinations and higher education; a survey of the literature, *Universities Quarterly*, 21, 292–340.

DALRYMPLE-CHAMPNEYS, W. (1955) The medical student through the ages, *Proc. roy. Soc. Med.*, 48, 789–98.

DANARAJ, T. J. (1966) University of Malaya Medical Centre, *Brit. J. med. Educ.*, 1, 62–8.

DARLEY, W. (1965) AAMC milestones in raising the standards of medical education, *J. med. Educ.*, 40, 321–8.

DAVIDSON, J. K., and THOMSON, G. O. B. (1970) Closed-circuit television in teaching diagnostic radiology, *Brit. J. med. Educ.*, 4, 23–8.

DAVIDSON, J. N. (1971) The role of the medically qualified preclinical teacher, *Scot. med. J.*, **16**, 241–6.

DAVIS, D. R. (1970) Behavioural science in the preclinical curriculum, *Brit. J. med. Educ.*, **4**, 194–7.

DENTON, E. J., and PHILLIPS, C. G. (1965) Memorandum of evidence on the medical curriculum submitted to the General Medical Council and the University Grants Committee by the Physiological Society, April, London.

DIAMENT, M. L., and GOLDSMITH, R. (1970) A simple automated method of marking multiple-choice questionnaires using a computer, *Brit. J. med. Educ.*, **4**, 53–5.

DICKINSON, W. R. (1953) Quoted from *Trans. Amer. clin. climat. Ass.*, **65**, 91.

DOMBAL, F. T. de, HARTLEY, J. R., and SLEEMAN, D. H. (1969) A computer-assisted system for learning clinical diagnosis, *Lancet*, **i**, 145–8.

DOMBAL, F. T. de, HORROCKS, J. C., STANILAND, J. R., and GILL, P. W. (1971) Simulation of clinical diagnosis; a comparative study, *Brit. med. J.*, **2**, 575–81.

DORST, S. (1947) The premedical program, *Cincinn. J. Med.*, **28**, 176–83.

DUDLEY, H. A. F. (1969) Objects of objective tests; a theoretical and experimental analysis, *Brit. J. med. Educ.*, **3**, 155–9.

DUDLEY, H. A. F. (1970) A first degree in clinical science, *Brit. J. med. Educ.*, **4**, 114–16.

DUNLOP, D. (1962) Medical education in Scotland, *Scot. med. J.*, **7**, 245–9.

EKEID, S. E. (1966) Studiosi vagantes: B.M.S.A. and student travel, *Brit. J. med. Educ.*, **1**, 52–7.

ELLIS, J. R. (1956a) Changes in medical education, *Lancet*, **i**, 813–18, 867–72.

ELLIS, J. R. (1956b) The tutorial system in medical schools, *Lancet*, **ii**, 375–8.

ELLIS, J. R. (1956c) The medical student, *J. med. Educ.*, **31**, 42–6.

ELLIS, J. R. (1965) Tomorrow's doctors, *Brit. med. J.*, **1**, 1571–7.

ELLIS, J. R. (1966a) A.S.M.E., *Brit. J. med. Educ.*, **1**, 2–6.

ELLIS, J. R. (1966b) The growth of science and the reform of the curriculum, in *The Evolution of Medical Education in Britain*, ed. Poynter, F. N. L., London.

ELLIS, J. R. (1967) Studying in depth in a clinical subject, *Brit. J. med. Educ.*, **1**, 94–8.

EYSENCK, H. J. (1953) *Uses and Abuses of Psychology*, Harmondsworth.

FLETCHER, S., and WATSON, A. A. (1968) Magnetic tape recording in the teaching of histopathology, *Brit. J. med. Educ.*, **2**, 278–82.

FLEXNER, A. (1910) *Medical Education in the United States and Canada*, A report to the Carnegie Foundation for the Advancement of Teaching, Bulletin No. 4, New York.

FLEXNER, A. (1912) *Medical Education in Europe*, New York.

FULTON, J. F. (1953) History of medical education, *Brit. med. J.*, **2**, 457–61.

GARRAWAY, W. M. (1969) British medical students in the U.S.A., *Brit. J. med. Educ.*, **3**, 215–20.

GEERTSMA, R. H., and CHAPMAN, J. E. (1967) The evaluation of medical students, *J. med. Educ.*, **42**, 938–48.

GENERAL MEDICAL COUNCIL (1967) *Recommendations as to Basic Medical Education*, General Medical Council, London.

GESELL, A. L., and ILG, F. (1949) *Infant and Child in the Culture of Today*, New York.

GIBSON, A. L. (1969) Second thoughts on multiple choice examinations, *Brit. J. med. Educ.*, **3**, 143–50.

GISH, O. (1970) British doctor migration 1962–67, *Brit. J. med. Educ.*, **4**, 279–88.

GOLDSTEIN, A. (1958) An enquiry into the value of rank grades in the medical course, *J. med. Educ.*, **33**, 193–200.

GRAHAM-LITTLE, E. (1939) The history of medical education in the last hundred years, *Med. Press*, **201**, 110–14.

GREENE, R. (1969) Are medical books too dear?, *Brit. med. J.*, **2**, 229.

GREULICH, W. W. (1953) In *Proceedings of First World Conference on Medical Education*, London, p. 231.

HACKETT, C. J. (1953) The teaching medical museum, *Med. biol. Ill.*, **3**, 146–57.

HARDEN, R. McG., LEVER, R., and WILSON, G. M. (1969) Two systems of marking objective examination questions, *Lancet*, **i**, 40–2.

HARRELL, G. T. (1968) Design of a medical school and its teaching hospital, *Brit. J. med. Educ.*, **2**, 252–64.

HARRIS, C. (1970) A teaching methods course in Liverpool for general practitioners, *Brit. J. med. Educ.*, **4**, 149–57.

HARRIS, H. (1971) Review of *Genes, Dreams and Realities*, by Burnet, M., *Brit. med. J.*, **3**, 712.

HARRISON, G. A., WEINER, J. S., TANNER, J. M., and BARNICOT, N. A. (1964) *Human Biology*, Oxford.

HAVARD, C. W. H. (1969) Are medical books too dear?, *Brit. med. J.*, **2**, 228.

HAWKINS, C. (1968) Bedside teaching, *Brit. med. J.*, **1**, 702–3.

HEALEY, J. E. (1969) A dilemma in medical education, *Surg. Gynec. Obstet.*, **128**, 1067–8.

HENN, T. R. (1951) The causes of failure in examinations, *Brit. med. J.*, **2**, 461–4.

HEYWOOD, J. (1969) In *Assessment of Undergraduate Performance*, Report of Conference at the University of London convened by the Committee of Vice-Chancellors and Principals and the Association of University Teachers, 27 March, London.

HILL, K. (1971) Preclinical salaries, *Brit. med. J.*, **3**, 116.

HINES, D. (1970) The application of anatomy and other basic medical sciences in general practice, *Brit. J. med. Educ.*, **4**, 145–8.

HOOPER, D. (1968) Behavioural science for preclinical students, *Lancet*, **ii**, 1293–5.

HOPSON, B. (1967) Lectures without tears, *The Guardian*, 23 March.

HUBBARD, J. P., and CLEMANS, W. V. (1961) *Multiple Choice Examinations in Medicine*, Philadelphia.

HUBBARD, W. N., and HOWARD, R. B. (1967) The educational environment in the large medical school, *J. med. Educ.*, **42**, 633–41.

HUBBLE, D. (1960) Medicine in its setting, *Lancet*, **i**, 1359–62.

HUSAK, T. (1968) M.C.Q. and the Membership, *Lancet*, **i**, 859–60.

ILLINGWORTH, C. (1968) The effect of scientific and technological advance on medicine and its implications for medical education, *J. med. Educ.*, **43**, 176–81.

IRONSIDE, W. (1963) *Magical Thinking, Modern Medicine and the Curriculum: An Inaugural Address*, University of Otago, Dunedin, New Zealand.

JACOBSON, E. D. (1967) Revolution in the medical curriculum, *J. med. Educ.*, **42**, 1081–6.

JASON, H. (1966) Sequential examinations in assessing the impact of a new medical curriculum, *J. med. Educ.*, **41** (Part 2), 18–24.

JASON, H. (1968) Self-instruction in medical education: principles, practice, proposals, *Brit. J. med. Educ.*, **2**, 278–82.

JEFFERYS, P. M. (1969) The teaching of community medicine in the undergraduate curriculum, *Brit. J. med. Educ.*, **3**, 176–84.

JOYCE, C. R. B., and HUDSON, L. (1968) Student style and teacher style: an experimental study, *Brit. J. med. Educ.*, **2**, 28–32.

JOYCE, C. R. B., and WEATHERALL, M. (1957) Controlled experiments in teaching, *Lancet*, **ii**, 402–7.

JOYCE, C. R. B. and WEATHERALL, M. (1959) Effective use of teaching time, *Lancet*, **i**, 568–71.

KELMAN, G. R. (1971) Preclinical salaries, *Brit. med. J.*, **3**, 537.

KEMP, T. A. (1968) The ecology of medical students, *Brit. J. med. Educ.*, **2**, 265–70.

KING, G. (1958) The medical school of the University of Western Australia, *J. med. Educ.*, **33**, 709–16.

KNOX, M. (1965) Address to the General Council of the University of St. Andrews, 26 June, St. Andrews.

LAST, J. M. (1968) How many doctors do we need?, *Lancet*, **ii**, 166–7.

LAUWERYS, J. A. (1950) Methods of education, *Brit. med. J.*, **2**, 471–4.

LENNON, G. G. (1971) Undergraduate medical education. Six years or five?, *Med. J. Aust.*, **1**, 1397–9.

LENNOX, B. (1967) Multiple choice, *Brit. J. med. Educ.*, **1**, 340–4.

LENNOX, B., and LEVER, R. (1970) Seminar on the machine marking of medical multiple choice question papers, *Brit. J. med. Educ.*, **4**, 219–27.

LEVIT, E. J. (1967) Use of the National Board 'Minitest' for evaluation of curricular change, *J. med. Educ.*, **42**, 930–4.

LIEBOW, A. (1956) Medicine taught as human biology, *Brit. med. J.*, **1**, 305–9.

LOGAN, R. (1969) The teaching of community medicine in the undergraduate curriculum, *Brit. J. med. Educ.*, **3**, 185–91.

McANDREW, G. M., DAWSON, A. A., and OGSTON, D. (1970) The under-graduate medical curriculum in retrospect, *Brit. J. med. Educ.*, **4**, 293–8.

McCARTHY, W. H. (1966) An assessment of the influence of cueing items in objective examinations, *J. med. Educ.*, **41**, 263–6.

McCARTHY, W. H. (1970) Improving large audience teaching: the 'pro-grammed' lecture, *Brit. J. med. Educ.*, **4**, 29–31.

McCARTHY, W. H., and GONNELLA, J. S. (1967) The simulated patient management problem; a technique for evaluating and teaching clinical competence, *Brit. J. med. Educ.*, **1**, 348–52.

McGUIRE, C. H. (1963) A process approach to the construction and analysis of medical examinations, *J. med. Educ.*, **38**, 556–63.

McGUIRE, C. H. (1965) The process approach to evaluation of medical curricula; theory and practice, in *Conference on Medical Education in South Africa, July 1964*, ed. Reid, J. V. O., and Wilmot, A. J., Natal University, Pietermaritzburg.

McGUIRE, C. H. (1966) The oral examination as a measure of professional competence, *J. med. Educ.*, **41**, 267–74.

MACKEITH, R. (1969) In *Education Conference, 1969*, British Medical Students' Association, BMA House, London.

MAIR, A. (1955) The medical curriculum; an opinion survey among Scottish graduates, *Brit. med. J.*, **2**, 526–34.

MALLESON, N. (1968) New textbooks for new education, in Book supple-ment, June 14th, *Med. News (N.Y.)*.

MARSHALL, M. S. (1951) The preclinical status, *J. med. Educ.*, **26**, 287–93.

MARSHALL, M. S. (1953) *Two Sides to a Teacher's Desk*, New York.

MARSHALL, M. S. (1954) What to do about grades, *J. Higher Educ.*, **25**, 263–8.

MARSHALL, M. S. (1956a) Objections to the objective objective, *Educational Forum*, March, 279–85.

MARSHALL, M. S. (1956b) Some trends and issues in medical education, *School and Society*, **83**, 179–83.

MARSHALL, M. S. (1958a) The structuring of examinations, *Educational Forum*, January, 139–46.

MARSHALL, M. S. (1958b) This thing called evaluation, *Educational Forum*, November, 41–53.

MARSHALL, M. S. (1963) The hydra of the campus, *Liberal Education*, **49**, 528–36.

MARSHALL, M. S. (1968) *Teaching Without Grades*, Oregon State Univer-sity, Corvallis, Oregon.

MARSHALL, M. S. (1969a) Lectures, Yes, *Phi Kappa Phi J.*, **49**, 14–20.

MARSHALL, M. S. (1969b) Academic anomaly, *Liberal Education*, **55**, 279–82.

MARTIN, B. F., *et al.* (1971) Preclinical salaries, *Brit. med. J.*, **4**, 237.

MARTIN, C. P. (1957) The place of anatomy in an expanding medical curriculum, *J. med. Educ.*, **32**, 215–27.

MARTIN, F. M., McPHERSON, F. M., and MAYO, P. R. (1967) A course in psychology and sociology for medical students, *Lancet*, ii, 411–13.

MEADOW, R. (1970) Personal view, *Brit. med. J.*, **2**, 704.

MEKIE, D. E. C. (1969) Master and apprentice, *J. roy. Coll. Surg. Edinb.*, **14**, 241–8.

MEREDITH, G. P. (1950) The art of lecturing, *Brit. med. J.*, **2**, 475–7.

MERSKEY, H. (1969) Some features of medical education in Great Britain during the first half of the nineteenth century, *Brit. J. med. Educ.*, **3**, 118–21.

MEYRICK, R. L. (1968) Closed circuit television in medicine, *Brit. J. med. Educ.*, **2**, 229–33.

MILLAR, M. (1962) Thoughts of a psychiatrist on medical education, *Scot. med. J.*, **7**, 507–11.

MILLER, G. E. (1962) An enquiry into medical teaching, *J. med. Educ.*, **37**, 185–91.

MILLER, G. E. (1969) The study of medical education, *Brit. J. med. Educ.*, **3**, 5–14.

MILLER, G. E. *et al.* (1961) *Teaching and Learning in Medical School*, Harvard University, Boston, Mass.

MILLER, H. (1966) Fifty years after Flexner, *Lancet*, **ii**, 647–54.

MILLER, H. (1971) Medical education and medical research, *Lancet*, **i**, 1–6.

MOLL, W. (1968) History of American medical education, *Brit. J. med. Educ.*, **2**, 173–81.

NETSKY, M. G. (1960) The teacher in the medical school, *J. med. Educ.*, **35**, 429–34.

NEWMAN, C. (1957) *The Evolution of Medical Education in the Nineteenth Century*, London.

NISBET, J. (1967) Courses on university teaching methods, *Universities Quarterly*, March, 186–98.

OGSTON, D., and McANDREW, G. M. (1967) Attitudes of patients to clinical teaching, *Brit. J. med. Educ.*, **1**, 316–19.

OLSON, I. A. (1970) Advantages and disadvantages of closed-circuit television in the teaching of large classes in preclinical medicine, *Brit. J. med. Educ.*, **4**, 312–15.

OSS, O. VAN (1971) What should we teach them?, *Proc. roy. Soc. Med.*, **64**, 600–1.

OWEN, S. G. (1966) *Electrocardiography*, London.

PARKINSON, C. N. (1965) *Parkinson's Law*, Harmondsworth.

PATTERSON, J. W. (1956) Western Reserve: interdepartmental and departmental teaching of medicine and biological science in four years, *J. med. Educ.*, **31**, 521–9.

PERRY, W. L. M. (1966) A study of medical student selection and performance in the Edinburgh medical school, *Brit. J. med. Educ.*, **1**, 16–24.

PICKERING, G. W. (1956) The purpose of medical education, *Brit. med. J.*, **2**, 113–16.

PICKERING, G. W. (1958) Medicine's challenge to the educator, *Brit. med. J.*, **2**, 1117–21.

PICKERING, G. W. (1959) A study of medical education in Great Britain, *J. med. Educ.*, **34**, 1139–46.

PICKERING, G. W. (1968) Some new issues in medical education, *Oxford med. Sch. Gaz.*, **20**, 95–105.

PICKERING, G. W. (1969) Postgraduate education and society: the lesson from medicine, *Brit. med. J.*, **3**, 375–8.

PICKERING, G. W. (1971) Science for pleasure or science for profit?, *Brit. med. J.*, **2**, 131–5.

PLATT, R. (1965) Thoughts on teaching medicine, *Brit. med. J.*, **2**, 551–2.

PLATT, R. (1967) Medical science; master or servant?, *Brit. med. J.*, **4**, 439–44.

POYNTER, F. N. L. (1966) Education and the General Medical Council, in *The Evolution of Medical Education in Britain*, ed. Poynter, F. N. L., London.

PRITCHARD, J. J. (1970) Soma without psyche, *Brit. J. med. Educ.*, **4**, 185–8.

PYKE, D. (1969) Are medical books too dear?, *Brit. med. J.*, **2**, 227.

QUILLIAM, T. A. (1968) Trends and prospects in technology-aided teaching in universities, in *Communication Media in Medicine*, B.I.S.F.A., London.

REPORT OF THE INTERDEPARTMENTAL COMMITTEE ON MEDICAL SCHOOLS (GOODENOUGH) (1944) London, H.M.S.O.

REPORT OF THE ROYAL COMMISSION ON UNIVERSITY EDUCATION IN LONDON (HALDANE) (1913) London, H.M.S.O.

REPORT OF THE ROYAL COMMISSION ON MEDICAL EDUCATION (TODD) (1968) London, H.M.S.O.

REPORT OF THE UNIVERSITY GRANTS COMMITTEE ON UNIVERSITY TEACHING METHODS (HALE) (1964) London, H.M.S.O.

ROBERTS, FF. (1948) *Medical Education*, London.

ROBERTS, K. B. (1967) The General Medical Council's Recommendations as to Basic Medical Education 1967, 2. The views of a teacher of physiology, *Brit. J. med. Educ.*, **1**, 239–41.

ROYAL COLLEGE OF PHYSICIANS (1944) *Report of the Royal College of Physicians of London Planning Committee on Medical Education*, Royal College of Physicians, London.

RUSSELL, D. (1968a) Personal view, *Brit. med. J.*, **2**, 248.

RUSSELL, D. (1968b) Personal view, *Brit. med. J.*, **2**, 800.

SANDERSON, P. H. (1969) The art of setting multiple-choice questions, *Lancet*, **ii**, 1291–4.

SAUNDERS, R. H. (1967) Use of a special examination designed with specific reference to curricular content, *J. med. Educ.*, **42**, 935–7.

SIMPSON, M. A., and MATTHEWS, T. (1968) *Report on Medical Education*, British Medical Students' Association, BMA House, London.

SINCLAIR, D. C. (1953a) Basic science, *Lancet*, **ii**, 463–7.

SINCLAIR, D. C. (1953b) Objective examination papers in the medical curriculum, *Lancet*, **ii**, 947–51.

SINCLAIR, D. C. (1955) *Medical Students and Medical Sciences*, London.

SINCLAIR, D. C. (1956a) The selection of medical students, *Univ. Leeds med. J.*, **5**, 51–3.

SINCLAIR, D. C. (1956b) The student textbook, *J. med. Educ.*, **31**, 697–705.

SINCLAIR, D. C. (1957a) British medical education and the General Medical Council, *J. med. Educ.*, **32**, 26–9.

SINCLAIR, D. C. (1957b) The London medical student's point of view, *J. med. Educ.*, **32**, 177–80.

SINCLAIR, D. C. (1957c) The place of anatomy in the medical curriculum, *Postgrad. med. J.*, **33**, 160–4.

SINCLAIR, D. C. (1957d) Medical education at Oxford, *J. med. Educ.*, **32**, 467–75.

SINCLAIR, D. C. (1958) A new medical curriculum, *Lancet*, **ii**, 430–4.

SINCLAIR, D. C. (1965a) An experiment in the teaching of anatomy, *J. med. Educ.*, **40**, 401–13.

SINCLAIR, D. C. (1965b) Preclinical teaching programme in the faculty of medicine, University of Western Australia, *Indian J. med. Educ.*, **5**, 1–10.

SINCLAIR, D. C. (1966) Anatomy in a changing curriculum, *Brit. med. Stud. J.*, **21**, 41–4.

SINCLAIR, D. C. (1972) Evaluation of a new medical curriculum (in preparation).

SINCLAIR, H. M., and ROBB-SMITH, A. H. T. (1950) *A History of the Teaching of Anatomy in Oxford*, Oxford.

SKANDAKIS, J. E., and GRAY, S. W. (1969) The very unpopular science, *Surg. Gynec. Obstet.*, **128**, 350.

SMART, I. H. M. (1971) *Notes on the Teaching of Anatomy at the University of Copenhagen and the Dental School at Aarhus*, Anatomy Department, University of Dundee.

SMITH, G. and WYLLIE, J. H. (1965) Use of closed-circuit television in teaching surgery to medical students, *Brit. med. J.*, **2**, 99–101.

SMITH, G., WYLLIE, J. H., FOOTE, A. V., and CARIDIS, D. T. (1966) Further studies on the use of closed-circuit television in teaching surgery to undergraduate medical students, *Brit. J. med. Educ.*, **1**, 40–2.

SOBIN, L. H. (1968) Self-instructive museum courses, *Brit. J. med. Educ.*, **2**, 278–82.

STOKES, J. F. (1967) Examining in the United States; the National Board of Examiners, *Brit. J. med. Educ.*, **1**, 320–9.

STRASSMAN, H. D., TAYLOR, D. D., and SCOLES, J. (1969) A new concept for a core medical curriculum, *J. med. Educ.*, **44**, 170–7.

TANNER, J. M. (1958) The place of human biology in medical education, *Lancet*, **i**, 1185–8.

THOMSON, A. P. D. (1966) A summary of the merits and demerits of the undergraduate training experienced by doctors now in practice in Central Africa, *Cent. Afr. J. Med.*, **12**, 184–91.

TIZARD, H. (1934) Presidential address to the Education Section of the British Association for the Advancement of Science, London.

TOWERS, B. (1969) Personal view, *Brit. med. J.*, **1**, 443.

TRETHOWAN, W. H. (1970) Assessment of Birmingham medical students, *Brit. med. J.*, **4**, 109–11.

UNIVERSITY GRANTS COMMITTEE (1968) *Enquiry into Student Progress*, London, H.M.S.O.

WALSHE, F. M. R. (1956) Medicine in the framework of the university, *Brit. med. J.*, **1**, 1441–4.

WALSHE, F. M. R. (1959) William Harvey upon Lord Chancellor Bacon, *Perspect. Biol. Med.*, **2**, 197–207.

WALKER, R. M. (1965) *Medical Education in Britain: A Rock Carling Fellowship Monograph*, Nuffield Provincial Hospitals Trust, London.

WALTON, H. J. (1966) *An Experimental Study of Effects on Medical Students of Three Methods of Teaching Psychiatry*, Ph.D. Thesis, Edinburgh (see *Brit. med. J.*, 1967, **2**, 124).

WALTON, H. J. (1968) Sex differences in ability and outlook of senior medical students, *Brit. J. med. Educ.*, **2**, 156–62.

WALTON, H. J., and DREWERY, J. (1967) The objective examination in the evaluation of medical students, *Brit. J. med. Educ.*, **1**, 255–64.

WALTON, H. J., DREWERY, J., and PHILLIPS, A. E. (1964) Typical medical students, *Brit. med. J.*, **2**, 744–8.

WHITEHEAD, R. (1952) Education by travel, *Lancet*, ii, 396–400.

WILLIAMS, B. (1969) Personal view, *Brit. med. J.*, **2**, 165.

WILLIAMS, P. C. (1965) Suggestions for speakers and standards for slides, *Inst. Biol. J.*, May.

WILLIAMSON, J. W. (1965) Assessing clinical judgement, *J. med. Educ.*, **40**, 180–7.

WILSON, G. M., HARDEN, R. McG., LEVER, R., ROBERTSON, J. I. S., and MACRITCHIE, J. (1969) Examination of clinical examiners, *Lancet*, **i**, 37–40.

WYMAN, J. B. (1971) What should we teach them?, *Proc. roy. Soc. Med.*, **64**, 604–6.

Index

Figures in bold type indicate extended treatment of subject referred to.